# Pain in the Joints

## Mission Statement of IASP Press®

IASP brings together scientists, clinicians, health care providers, and policy makers to stimulate and support the study of pain and to translate that knowledge into improved pain relief worldwide. IASP Press publishes timely, high-quality, and reasonably priced books relating to pain research and treatment.

# Pain in the Joints

**Lars Arendt-Nielsen, PhD, DMSc**
Professor
Center for Sensory-Motor Interaction (SMI)
Department of Health Science and Technology
Faculty of Medicine
Aalborg University
Aalborg, Denmark

**Serge Perrot, MD, PhD**
Professor
Centre d'Evaluation et de Traitement de la Douleur
Université Paris Descartes
INSERM U 987
Paris, France

Wolters Kluwer
Philadelphia • Baltimore • New York • London
Buenos Aires • Hong Kong • Sydney • Tokyo

International Association for the Study of Pain
IASP®
*Working together for pain relief*

*Acquisitions Editor*: Keith Donnellan
*Product Development Editor*: Lauren Pecarich
*Production Project Manager*: David Orzechowski
*Design Coordinator*: Holly McLaughlin
*Manufacturing Coordinator*: Beth Welsh
*Marketing Manager*: Dan Dressler
*Prepress Vendor*: S4Carlisle Publishing Services



9 8 7 6 5 4 3 2 1

Printed in China

**Library of Congress Cataloging-in-Publication Data**

Names: Arendt-Nielsen, Lars, 1958- editor. | Perrot, Serge, 1960- editor. | International Association for the Study of Pain, issuing body.
Title: Pain in the joints / [edited by] Lars Arendt-Nielsen, Serge Perrot.
Description: First edition. | Philadelphia : Wolters Kluwer Health, [2017] | Includes bibliographical references and index.
Identifiers: LCCN 2016020392 | ISBN 9781496353627
Subjects: | MESH: Arthralgia—physiopathology | Arthralgia—therapy | Chronic pain
Classification: LCC RB127.5.C48 | NLM WE 304 | DDC 616/.0472—dc23 LC record available at https://lccn.loc.gov/2016020392



LWW.com

CCS0716

# CONTRIBUTORS


*Lars Arendt-Nielsen, PhD, DMSc*
Professor
Center for Sensory-Motor Interaction (SMI)
Department of Health Science and Technology
Faculty of Medicine
Aalborg University
Aalborg, Denmark

*Sadaf Ashraf, PhD*
Postdoctoral Fellow
Arthritis Research UK Pain Centre
University of Nottingham
School of Pharmacy
University Park
Nottingham, United Kingdom

*Pierre Beaulieu, MD, PhD, FRCA*
Professor
Department of Anesthesiology and Pharmacology
Faculty of Medicine
University of Montreal
Montreal, Québec, Canada

*Lisa C. Carlesso, PT, PhD*
Assistant Professor
School of Rehabilitation
Faculty of Medicine
University of Montreal
Orthopaedic Clinical Research Unit
Maisonneuve-Rosemont Hospital Research Centre
Montreal, Québec, Canada

*Victoria Chapman, PhD*
Professor
Arthritis Research UK Pain Centre
University of Nottingham
School of Biomedical Sciences
Queen's Medical Centre
Nottingham, United Kingdom

*Xavier Chevalier, MD, PhD*
Head
Department of Rheumatology
Henri Mondor Hospital
Créteil, France

*Jacqui Clinch, MBBS, MRCP*
Consultant Paediatric Rheumatologist
Bristol Royal Hospital for Children
Lead Consultant
Adolescent Pain Management Service
Bath Centre for Pain Services
Bath, Avon, United Kingdom

*Aileen M. Davis, PT, PhD*
Senior Scientist
Health Care and Outcomes Research
Toronto Western Research Institute
University Health Network
Professor
Department of Physical Therapy
Institute of Rehabilitation Science
Institute of Health, Policy, Management, and Evaluation
University of Toronto
Toronto, Ontario, Canada

*Florent Eymard, MD*
Rheumatologist
Department of Rheumatology
Henri Mondor Hospital
Cretéil, France

*Kerstin Gerhold, MD, PhD, MSc*
Head
Section of Pediatric Rheumatology
Department of Pediatrics and Child Health
Assistant Professor of Pediatrics
University of Manitoba
Winnipeg, Manitoba, Canada

*Dorien Goubert, MSc*
Research Fellow
Pain in Motion International Research Group
Department of Rehabilitation Sciences and Physiotherapy
Faculty of Medicine and Health Sciences
Ghent University
Ghent, Belgium

*Margaret E. Gruen, DVM, MVPH, PhD*
Diplomate
American College of Veterinary Behavior
Comparative Pain Research Program
North Carolina State University College of Veterinary Medicine
Raleigh, North Carolina

*Ali Guermazi, MD, PhD*
Professor of Radiology
Quantitative Imaging Center (QIC)
Department of Radiology
Boston University School of Medicine
Boston, Massachusetts

*Gillian A. Hawker, MD, MSc*
Professor
Department of Medicine
Institute for Health Policy, Management and Evaluation
University of Toronto
Senior Scientist
Women's College Research Institute
Women's College Hospital
Adjunct Scientist
Institute for Clinical Evaluative Sciences
Toronto, Ontario, Canada

*Yves Henrotin, PhD*
Professor
Department of Pathology
Physical Therapy and Rehabilitation
Director
Bone and Cartilage Research Unit
University of Liège (Belgium)
Head
Department of Physical Therapy and Rehabilitation
Princess Paola Hospital
Marche-en-Famenne, Belgium

*Jacqueline R. Hochman, BSc, MD, FRCPC, MSc*
Assistant Professor
Division of Rheumatology
Department of Medicine
Women's College Hospital
University of Toronto
Toronto, Ontario, Canada

*Tatsunori Ikemoto, MD, PhD*
Assistant Professor
Multidisciplinary Pain Center
Institute of Physical Fitness, Sports Medicine, and Rehabilitation
Aichi Medical University
Nagakute, Aichi, Japan

*John F. Innes, BVSc, PhD, CertVR, DSAS(orth), MRCVS*
Professor
Clinical Director
ChesterGates Veterinary Specialists
Chester, Cheshire, United Kingdom
Referrals Director
CVS(UK) Limited
Honorary Professor
Veterinary School
University of Liverpool
Liverpool, Merseyside, United Kingdom

*Masashi Izumi, MD, PhD*
Research Associate
Department of Orthopaedic Surgery
Kochi Medical School
Kochi University
Nankoku, Kochi, Japan

*Motohiro Kawasaki, MD, PhD*
Assistant Professor
Department of Orthopaedic Surgery
Kochi Medical School
Kochi University
Nankoku, Kochi, Japan

*B. Duncan X. Lascelles, BSc, BVSc, PhD, MRCVS, CertVA, DSAS(ST), DECVS, DACVS*
Professor
Department of Surgery and Pain Management
Comparative Pain Research Program
North Carolina State University College of Veterinary Medicine
Raleigh, North Carolina
Center for Pain Research and Innovation
UNC Chapel Hill, North Carolina

*Mira Meeus, PhD*
Professor
Faculty of Medicine and Health Science
University of Antwerp
Wilrijk, Belgium

*Tuhina Neogi, MD, PhD, FRCPC*
Professor of Medicine and Epidemiology
Sections of Clinical Epidemiology Unit and Rheumatology
Department of Medicine
Boston University School of Medicine
Department of Epidemiology
Boston University School of Public Health
Boston, Massachusetts

*John Nijs, PhD*
Professor
Pain in Motion International Research Group
Department of Physiotherapy
Human Physiology and Anatomy
Faculty of Physical Education and Physiotherapy
Vrije Universiteit Brussel
Brussels, Belgium

*Tomohiko Nishigami, PhD*
Associate Professor
Department of Physical Therapy
Konan-Women's University
Kobe, Osaka Bay, Japan

*Yoji Osako, PhD*
Associate Professor
Department of Neurobiology and Anatomy
Kochi Medical School
Kochi University
Nankoku, Kochi, Japan

*Serge Perrot, MD, PhD*
Professor
Centre d'Evaluation et de Traitement de la Douleur
Université Paris Descartes
INSERM U 987
Paris, France

*Kristian Kjær Petersen, MSc, PhD*
Postdoctoral Fellow
Center for Sensory-Motor Interaction (SMI)
Faculty of Medicine
Department of Health Science and Technology
Aalborg University
Aalborg, Denmark

*Stephan Reichenbach, MD, MSc*
Associate Professor
Department of Rheumatology, Immunology, and Allergology
Faculty of Medicine
University of Bern
Bern, Switzerland

*Frank W. Roemer, MD*
Associate Professor
Co-Director
Quantitative Imaging Center (QIC)
Department of Radiology
University of Erlangen-Nuremberg
Boston University School of Medicine
Boston Imaging Core Lab
Boston, Massachusetts

*Ewa M. Roos, PT, PhD*
Professor and Head
Research Unit for Musculoskeletal Function and Physiotherapy
Institute of Sports Science and Clinical Biomechanics
University of Southern Denmark
Odense, Denmark

*Devi Rani Sagar, PhD*
Postdoctoral Fellow
Arthritis Research UK Pain Centre
University of Nottingham
School of Biomedical Sciences
Queen's Medical Centre
Nottingham, United Kingdom

*Hans-Georg Schaible, MD*
Professor
Institute of Physiology/Neurophysiology
Jena University Hospital
Friedrich Schiller University of Jena
Jena, Germany

*Søren T. Skou, PT, PhD*
Postdoctoral Fellow
Research Unit for Musculoskeletal Function and Physiotherapy
Institute of Sports Science and Clinical Biomechanics
University of Southern Denmark
Odense, Denmark

*Tomoko Tetsunaga, MD, PhD*
Research Associate
Department of Orthopaedic Surgery
Graduate School of Medicine, Dentistry, and Pharmaceutical Sciences
Okayama University
Okayama, Japan

*Takahiro Ushida, MD, PhD*
Professor and Director
Multidisciplinary Pain Center
Director
Institute of Physical Fitness, Sports Medicine, and Rehabilitation
Aichi Medical University
Nagakute, Aichi, Japan

*Suzie Van Noten, PhD*
Predoctoral Research Fellow
Faculty of Medicine and Health Sciences
University of Antwerp
Wilrijk, Belgium

*Pascale Vergne-Salle, MD, PhD*
Professor
Department of Therapeutics
Service de Rhumatologie
Centre de la douleur
University Hospital of Limoges
Limoges, France

*Carl L. von Baeyer, PhD*
Professor Emeritus
Department of Psychology
Associate Member in Pediatrics
University of Saskatchewan
Saskatoon, Saskatchewan, Canada
Professor
Department of Clinical Health Psychology, Pediatrics, and Child Health
Faculty of Medicine
University of Manitoba
Winnipeg, Manitoba, Canada

*David A. Walsh, FRCP, PhD*
Professor
Department of Rheumatology
Director
Arthritis Research UK Pain Centre
University of Nottingham
Nottingham, United Kingdom

# PREFACE

IASP decided to focus the Global Year 2016 on joint pain because it is a substantially growing and complex problem that affects millions of people worldwide and is a major socioeconomic burden. As part of the activities in the Global Year against Joint Pain 2016, this book has been published with leading experts in this field as authors.

Musculoskeletal pain, including joint pain, is the major cause of chronic pain. Chronic pain caused by joint problems is assumed to further increase in future because of demographic and lifestyle changes. Joint pain is complex and far-reaching and is related to many different local and systemic diseases. A key feature of many joint pain problems is the lack of association between joint damage and the pain intensity felt by the patient, and hence other mechanisms (such as sensitization) may play a role. Another key feature is the importance of exercise and movement in joint pain pathophysiology, but also in its management. Despite the wide-ranging conditions and symptoms, different types of joint pain may, therefore, share similar underlying mechanisms, manifestations, and potential treatments. A translational pain research approach is important in this area and is reflected in the book.

Several key issues on joint pain have been identified:

- Treatment for joint pain is difficult as medication options are generally limited and not safe.
- Nonpharmacological approaches may be an option in selected patients.
- There are very few specific assessment tools for joint pain.
- Local and spreading sensitization seems prominent, and quantitative assessment is essential.
- Joint pain is characterized by different kinds of pain: at rest and on movement (provoked), with different mechanisms involved.
- Expansion of neuronal receptive fields in animals and expansion of pain areas in patients are examples of translational mechanisms.

- It is generally difficult for clinicians to identify links between imaging and the patient's actual pain, which makes joint pain especially challenging to understand, and hence the pain is often underestimated by the clinicians.
- Surgery (e.g., joint replacement) may in some cases not resolve the pain problem, and understanding of this phenomenon is important.

Beyond the suffering and discomfort associated with various types of joint pain, there are huge financial and other costs linked to this problem, including medical care expenses, lost work days, and diminished quality and productivity in patients' work and personal lives. Throughout the world, the numerous challenges surrounding joint pain are on the rise because of a number of accelerating factors and trends, such as:

- Aging populations
- Sedentary lifestyles
- Increasing incidence of obesity

This book on joint pain is aimed at providing a comprehensive overview of the pain problems, how to assess joint pain, mechanisms involved, and treatment options. It addresses the general concepts of the diagnostic and therapeutic challenges.

The book is not only of interest to pain scientists, but is also useful to clinicians involved in perioperative care and the management of chronic pain in general. The book also deals with the basic science of joint pain and aims to translate this into a better understanding of clinical joint pain conditions. Translational aspects from neurophysiology to genetics—investigating the pathophysiology of ongoing nociception, pain persistence, and chronic pain development also provides an interest for basic scientists.

With this book we have tried to reach out to different clinical disciplines involved in joint pain such as orthopedic surgeons, rheumatologists, pain specialists, and anaesthesiologists, but also to general practitioners, internists, neurologists, psychologists, and psychiatrists, who face the task of managing the long-term consequences of chronic joint pain.

The editorial process has been a pleasure, with many people devoting a lot of time to the book project. Obviously, this book would not have been possible without the authors, who are sincerely acknowledged for their enthusiastic contributions, high-quality manuscripts, and for meeting deadlines. Susanne Nielsen Lundis, Aalborg University, Denmark, has been incredibly important for keeping us all on track and liaised with the IASP Press, and we are very thankful for her continued help and dedication. We are also thankful to Editor-in-Chief Maria Adele Giamberardino and her staff at IASP Press.

We sincerely hope you will enjoy reading this book, and any feedback is highly appreciated.

*Lars Arendt-Nielsen*
*Serge Perrot*

# CONTENTS

# Pain in the Joints

CHAPTER 1

# Joint Pain Epidemiology

*Tuhina Neogi*

Pain is the most common symptom that leads individuals to seek medical attention; the most common type of chronic pain worldwide is musculoskeletal pain, especially joint and back pain (Fig. 1-1). The most common cause of joint pain is related to arthritis, of which there are numerous types. Joint pain is not only a complaint for which patients commonly seek medical attention, but it is also one of the leading causes of disability.

## PREVALENCE OF JOINT PAIN AND ARTHRITIS

Joint pain increases with age, and is generally more prevalent among women than men. It is also positively associated with body mass. Approximately one-third of adults with joint pain rate it as severe. The Global Burden of Disease Study 2010 found that musculoskeletal conditions collectively affect >2.9 billion people, and that prevalence has increased by 44.7% since 1990, with knee osteoarthritis (OA) being the most common joint condition [22] (Fig. 1-2). However, this prevalence and the relative proportions of the various conditions are likely underestimated as a number of diseases are not systematically surveyed in many countries. In a community-dwelling cohort of adults in Framingham, MA, who were unselected for any pain complaints, the most common site of pain, aching, or stiffness on most days was the back;

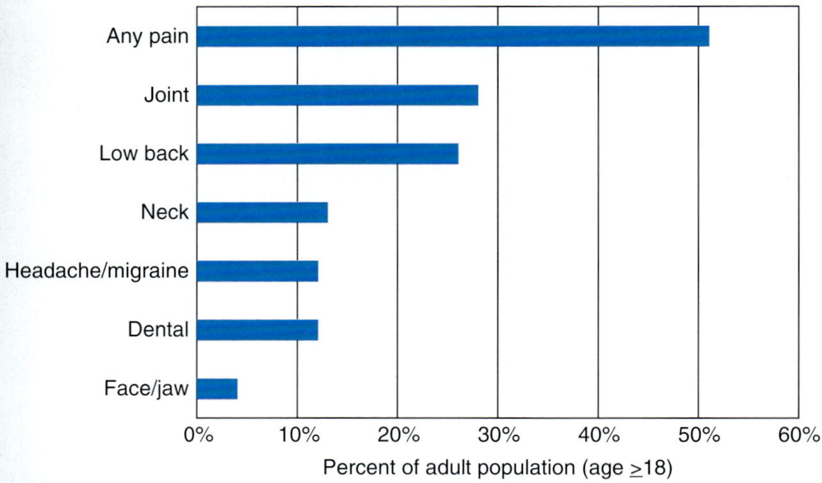


**FIGURE 1-1** Prevalence of pain at selected body sites. (From Pleis and Lucas [19].)

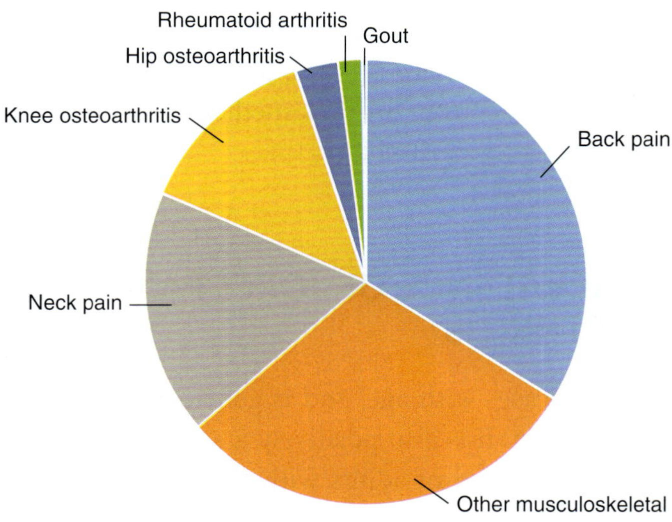


**FIGURE 1-2** Relative prevalence of common musculoskeletal conditions.(From March et al. [13].)

the knee was the most common joint site (Fig. 1-3). Only the elbow had a prevalence of less than 10% for pain, aching, or stiffness on most days; most other joint sites were in the 15–20% prevalence range. It should be noted that the hip and shoulder were also quite common, with a similar prevalence to that of neck pain.

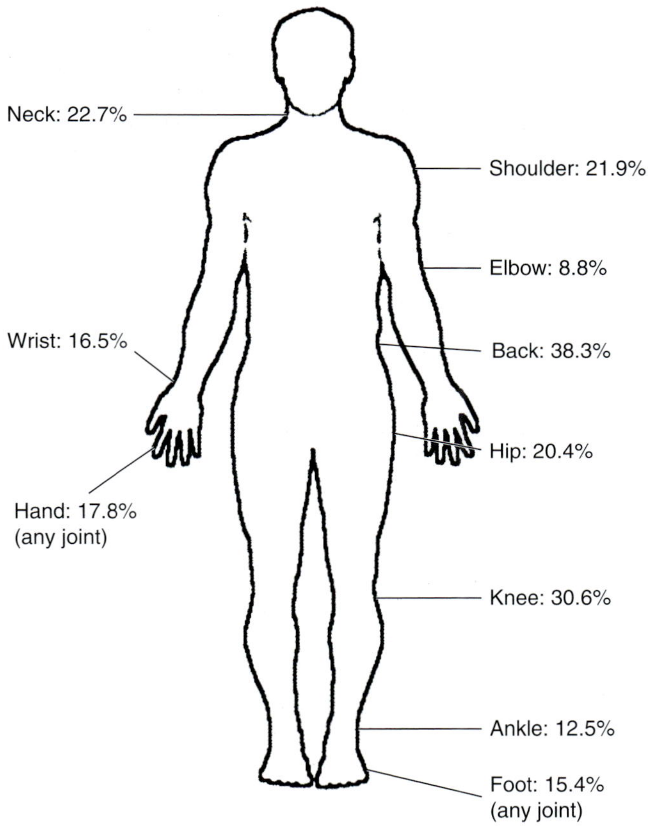


**FIGURE 1-3** Prevalence of pain in different body regions in a community-dwelling cohort in the United States (Framingham, MA).

In the United States, according to data from the National Health Interview Survey for the period 2010–2012, an estimated 52.5 million (22.7%) of adults self-reported doctor-diagnosed arthritis; this is approximately twice the number of American adults that have all types of heart disease (11.5%), and two-and-a-half times as many as those that have diabetes (8.8%) [21]. Further, 28.2% of adults (67 million) have chronic joint pain, and 22.7 million (9.8%) have arthritis-attributable activity limitation. It is estimated that by the year 2030, 67 million—one in every four American adults—will have doctor-diagnosed arthritis, two-thirds of whom will be women [2]. These future trends are likely to be conservative as they ignore trends in obesity; the worldwide prevalence of obesity has doubled between 1980 and 2014. The predicted increase in the prevalence of arthritis is particularly troubling as arthritis or other rheumatic conditions is already the leading cause of disability among American adults, accounting for 19% of all causes of disability based on U.S. Census data analyzed by the Centers of Disease Control and Prevention [6].

In Europe, 22% of the population has experienced long-term muscle, bone, and joint problems such as arthritis or other rheumatic conditions according to a 2007 European Commission Eurobarometer Survey [4]. Activity-limiting pain was reported in 18–46% of European countries; chronic musculoskeletal pain was reported in 13–33% of countries. Further, 32% of all respondents reported that they experienced muscle, joint, neck, or back pain that affected their activities of daily living, and 25% reported having experienced chronic restrictive musculoskeletal pain at some point in their life.

## EPIDEMIOLOGY OF SPECIFIC CONDITIONS CONTRIBUTING TO JOINT PAIN

### Osteoarthritis

Much of the worldwide experience of joint pain is due to OA, which is the most common form of arthritis, accounting for more disability among the elderly than any other disease. The disease involves the whole joint, is related to maladaptive repair responses resulting in pathologic changes in numerous joint tissues, and increases in prevalence with age. Major risk factors include obesity and joint injury, in addition to age. This disease has a higher prevalence among women than men. Not all individuals with radiographically evident disease experience pain. Symptomatic OA generally affects 10–15% of populations worldwide, with 27 million affected in the United States [10] and 8.75 million affected in the United Kingdom [1]. Data from the European Health Interview Surveys in seven countries demonstrated wide variation in prevalence of doctor-diagnosed OA, ranging from 5% to 25% (age-standardized range 3–18%) [4]. The knee, hand, and hip are common sites of OA, with the knee typically being considered to be the most common, particularly with regard to symptoms. About 30% of U.S. adults report some form of joint pain within the preceding 30 days, with the knee joint being the most common site. The knee is also the most common site of joint complaint restricting daily activity in European adults, after back pain. In general, the knee is the most common site of joint pain regardless of age, gender, or race. Of note, the last 20 years have seen an increase in prevalence of knee pain as well as of symptomatic knee OA, but not of radiographic knee OA itself; obesity only partially explained the increase in prevalence of knee pain [18].

## Back and Neck Pain

Although low back and neck pain are not traditionally thought of as joint pain conditions, they are highly prevalent and disabling, accounting for 16.8% of all causes of disability in the United States, where they are the second most common cause of disability after arthritis or other rheumatic conditions [6]. In Europe, chronic pain in the low back, upper back, and neck accounts for 20% of musculoskeletal pain that restricted daily activity [4]. These axial pain conditions can be related to osteoarthritic changes in the spine, although the etiology of low back and neck pain is multifactorial and not necessarily related to arthritis. Their heterogeneous nature is reflected in their reported point prevalence, ranging from 8% to 39% of the population for back pain, and from 6% to 39% for neck pain. Lifetime prevalence of back pain has been reported to vary from 60% to 85%; that of neck pain ranges from 14% to 71%. Most recent estimates from the Global Burden of Disease Study 2010 reported a point prevalence of 9.4% and 4.9% for low back and neck pain, respectively [7, 8]. Many people will experience one or more episodes of low back and/or neck pain in their lives.

## Gout

Gout, a crystal-related arthritis, is now the most common form of inflammatory arthritis, and is related to hyperuricemia. It is characterized by acute painful flares that can eventually become a chronic arthritis. Many patients describe their gout attacks as the most painful experience of their lives, worse than childbirth or a gunshot. Gout presently affects 1–4% of various populations around the world, with some populations, such as those of Maori ancestry, having a higher prevalence (6%) [17]. This variation in prevalence is related to the prevalence of associated comorbidities and risk factors, as well as genetics. The incidence and prevalence of gout have been rising over the recent decades, a trend thought to be related to the rise in obesity and adoption of less healthy diets (e.g., a Western diet) and less healthy lifestyles. Individuals with gout have a high burden of comorbidities, including metabolic syndrome, cardiovascular disease, and renal disease, among others.

## Rheumatoid Arthritis

Rheumatoid arthritis, the most common form of an autoimmune systemic inflammatory arthritis, is characterized by a typically symmetric polyarthritis with joint pain, swelling, and substantial morning stiffness. Rheumatoid arthritis affects less than 1% of populations worldwide [5]. Smoking is one of the strongest modifiable risk factors that have been identified. Individuals with rheumatoid arthritis have a higher risk of major adverse cardiovascular events independent of other traditional risk factors, as well as a higher risk of lymphoma and infections, which are thought to be related to both the degree of systemic inflammation and use of immunosuppressant drugs.

## Psoriatic Arthritis

Psoriatic arthritis is a chronic inflammatory arthritis associated with psoriasis, but can also occur in people without skin psoriasis. The inflammatory arthritis often follows the onset of skin psoriasis, but can also precede it, and affects peripheral joints, axial joints, or both. Psoriatic arthritis is a type of seronegative spondyloarthritis, which is a family of diseases that share common clinical features. The prevalence of psoriatic arthritis is 0.1–0.25% in the general population, and 6–11%

among people with psoriasis. As with patients suffering from other inflammatory arthritis conditions such as rheumatoid arthritis, those with psoriatic arthritis have an increased risk of cardiovascular disease.

### Juvenile Idiopathic Arthritis

Juvenile idiopathic arthritis is an umbrella term for the several types of inflammatory arthritis conditions that occur in childhood, with onset prior to age 16. Juvenile idiopathic arthritis is one of the more common chronic diseases of childhood. The worldwide prevalence of juvenile idiopathic arthritis is reported as 0.07–4.01 per 1000 children [11] It is estimated that 294,000 American children in the early 2000 era had a significant pediatric arthritis or other rheumatologic condition [20]. Juvenile idiopathic arthritis impacts not only childhood, but also adulthood; approximately 30% of individuals with juvenile idiopathic arthritis have significant functional limitations 10 or more years after its onset.

## CONSEQUENCES OF JOINT PAIN

### Disability

Musculoskeletal disorders are now the second leading cause of disability in terms of years lived with disability. They are also the fourth leading cause of total burden of disease in terms of disability-adjusted life-years as a time-based measure of health that considers both years of life lost as a result of premature mortality and years lived with disability [15, 22]. Given that most of these diseases are generally not fatal, the burden of disease reflects a substantial amount of disability over the lifetime of individuals. More specifically, low back pain itself ranked first, neck pain fourth, OA eleventh, and other musculoskeletal disorders ranked sixth in the Global Burden of Disease Study. These effects were fairly consistent through the different geographic regions. Thus, worldwide, joint pain and other musculoskeletal conditions represent a substantial public health burden. In addition to contributing to pain, these conditions are associated with functional limitations, participation restrictions, and disability. Further, some arthritis conditions have been associated with increased mortality, directly related to the underlying arthritis, the associated comorbidities, adverse outcomes, or to adverse events related to medications.

## Health Care Resource Utilization and Other Economic Impacts

The economic impact of joint pain is also substantial. The total costs attributable to arthritis and other rheumatic conditions in the United States in 2003 was ~$128 billion, or 1.2% of the 2003 U.S. gross domestic product. Of this, $80.8 billion accounted for direct costs, and $47 billion for indirect costs (e.g., lost earnings) [23]. Further, overall medical expenditures for individuals with arthritis were estimated to be $353 billion in 2005, reflecting the substantial comorbidities individuals with arthritis also suffer from, which add to the medical and economic burden of disease [3]. Arthritis-related conditions accounted for the largest increase in health care expenditures in the United States from 1996 to 2011 (192%), according to the Medical Expenditures Panel Survey. The mean per-person total direct costs in 2011 U.S. dollars for arthritis and joint pain in the United States were $9556 for the years 2009–2011; the total aggregate direct costs were $580.9 billion. The total aggregate costs (direct and indirect) for four selected musculoskeletal conditions are shown relative to their prevalence in the population in Fig. 1-4. For pediatric juvenile idiopathic arthritis and other pediatric rheumatologic conditions, total hospital charges in 2012 were $4.45 billion for those age 17 years and younger, according to the Healthcare Cost and Utilization Project Kids' Inpatient Database by the U.S. Agency for Healthcare Research and Quality.

Across the European Union, musculoskeletal conditions are among the largest diagnostic groups in terms of health care expenditures. In the United Kingdom, the estimated cost of general practitioner consultations for musculoskeletal conditions in 2003 was £1.34 million, second only to cardiorespiratory conditions. In Germany, the cost of diseases of the musculoskeletal system was €28.5 billion in 2008, accounting for more than 11% of the total illness costs that year.

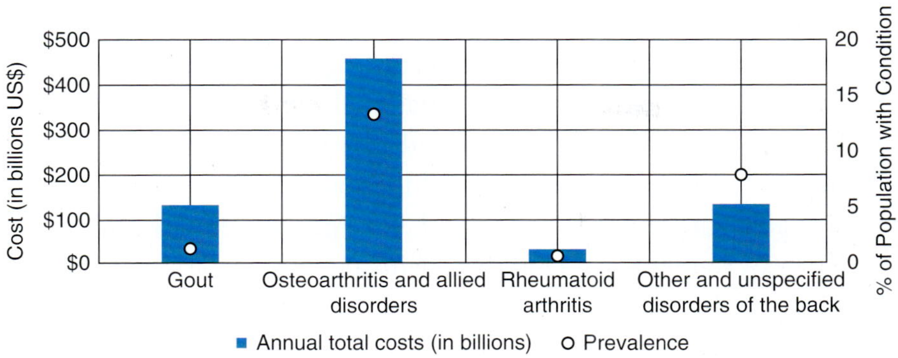


**FIGURE 1-4** Aggregate total costs for selected musculoskeletal diseases in the United States, 2008–2011. Dollar values reported are an average across the 4 years. (Medical Expenditures Panel Survey [MEPS] et al. [14].)

The productivity costs to the economy add further to these costs, in the form of absences from work, being less productive at work, and early retirement due to joint pain. Approximately 15% of American adults with joint pain report being unable to work; a similar percentage (15–18%) of adults with back or neck pain also report being unable to work. This figure increases to approximately 20% for those with arthritis.

In addition to work-related costs and health care resource utilization costs in terms of investigations, outpatient appointments, and hospitalizations, other health care impacts of joint pain include frequent use of analgesics. Approximately one-fifth of adults with joint pain report using nonprescription or prescription non-narcotic analgesics regularly and one-quarter report using prescription analgesics over the previous month [16]. These percentages are similar for back and neck pain, but increase to 37% for those with arthritis using a prescription analgesic drug in the previous month, and to 31% using nonprescription or prescription non-narcotic analgesics frequently in the previous month.

Another major economic impact is the rising number of joint replacements performed. Most (97%) knee replacement surgeries are performed for OA. In the United States alone, 4.7 million and 2.55 million adults in 2010 were living with a knee and hip arthroplasty, respectively, representing approximately 2% of the population, numbers that are similar to those living with a stroke or myocardial infarction

[12]. In that year (2010), 719,000 knee arthroplasties and 332,000 hip arthroplasties were performed, according to the National Hospital Discharge Survey. A survey of 10 national databases (Canada, Finland, France, Germany, Italy, Netherlands, Portugal, Spain, Switzerland, and the United States) as well as an additional eight countries with publicly available data (Australia, England and Wales, Denmark, New Zealand, Norway, Romania, and Sweden), with a total population of 755 million, reported that the median rate of total knee replacement was 149 procedures per 100,000, ranging from 8.8 (Romania) to 234 (United States) procedures per 100,000 population (Table 1-1), and the rates continue to rise [9]. These high rates of joint replacement surgery reflect the fact that there are no proven therapies to prevent or halt OA, with surgery being considered the definitive therapy for this condition.

TABLE 1-1 **International Utilization of Total Knee Replacement Procedures [9]**

| Country | Primary Total Knee Procedures/100,000 Population |
|---|---|
| Australia* (2008) | 165.5 |
| Canada (2008) | 143.7 |
| Denmark* (2008) | 143.3 |
| England and Wales* (2009/10) | 144.6 |
| Finland (2009) | 177.5 |
| France (2007) | 98.1 |
| Germany (2008) | 188.3 |
| Italy (2008) | 94.7 |
| Netherlands (2007)[†] | 121.2 |
| New Zealand* (2009) | 142.4 |
| Norway* (2008) | 84.8 |
| Portugal (2008) | 55.4 |
| Romania* (2009) | 8.6 |
| Scotland* (2009) | 135 |
| Spain (2008) | 82.9 |
| Sweden* (2008) | 111.6 |
| Switzerland (2008) | 176.8 |
| United States (2008) | 213.3 |

*From publicly available registries.

[†]This figure represents both primary and revision total knee procedures.

## CONCLUSION

In summary, joint pain is highly prevalent, disabling, and economically costly to societies worldwide. Many of these conditions do not have effective therapies, and for those that do, patients are often not adequately managed with existing therapies. The high prevalence and impact of these diseases on the patient and on society should be taken as a call to arms to find or improve effective strategies to help the millions suffering from joint pain around the world.

### REFERENCES


1. Arthritis Research UK. Osteoarthritis in general practice. London: Arthritis Research UK; 2013.
2. Barbour KE, Helmick CG, Theis KA, Murphy LB, Hootman JM, Brady TJ, Cheng YJ. Prevalence of doctor-diagnosed arthritis and arthritis-attributable activity limitation—United States, 2010–2012. MMWR Morb Mortal Wkly Rep 2013;62:869–73.
3. Cisternas MG, Murphy LB, Yelin EH, Foreman AJ, Pasta DJ, Helmick CG. Trends in medical care expenditures of US adults with arthritis and other rheumatic conditions 1997 to 2005. J Rheumatol 2009;36:2531–8.
4. European Musculoskeletal Surveillance and Information Network. Musculoskeletal health status in Europe. Accessed November 13 at www.eumusc.net/workpackages_wp4.cfm.
5. Gibofsky A. Overview of epidemiology, pathophysiology, and diagnosis of rheumatoid arthritis. Am J Manag Care 2012;18:S295–302.
6. Hootman JM, Brault MW, Helmick CG, Theis KA, Armour BS. Prevalence and most common causes of disability among adults—United States, 2005. MMWR Morb Mortal Wkly Rep 2009;58:421–26.
7. Hoy D, March L, Brooks P, Blyth F, Woolf A, Bain C, Williams G, Smith E, Vos T, Barendregt J, et al. The global burden of low back pain: estimates from the Global Burden of Disease 2010 study. Ann Rheum Dis 2014;73:968–74.
8. Hoy D, March L, Woolf A, Blyth F, Brooks P, Smith E, Vos T, Barendregt J, Blore J, Murray C, et al. The global burden of neck pain: estimates from the Global Burden of Disease 2010 study. Ann Rheum Dis 2014;73:1309–15.
9. Kurtz SM, Ong KL, Lau E, Widmer M, Maravic M, Gomez-Barrena E, de Pina Mde F, Manno V, Torre M, Walter WL, et al. International survey of primary and revision total knee replacement. Int Orthop 2011;35:1783–9.
10. Lawrence RC, Felson DT, Helmick CG, Arnold LM, Choi H, Deyo RA, Gabriel S, Hirsch R, Hochberg MC, Hunder GG, et al. Estimates of the prevalence of arthritis and other rheumatic conditions in the United States. Part II. Arthritis Rheum 2008;58:26–35.

11. Manners PJ, Bower C. Worldwide prevalence of juvenile arthritis why does it vary so much? J Rheumatol 2002;29:1520–30.
12. Maradit Kremers H, Larson DR, Crowson CS, Kremers WK, Washington RE, Steiner CA, Jiranek WA, Berry DJ. Prevalence of total hip and knee replacement in the United States. J Bone Joint Surg Am 2015;97:1386–97.
13. March L, Smith EUR, Hoy DG, Cross MJ, Sanchez-Riera L, Blyth F, Buchbinder R, Vos T, Woolf AD. Burden of disability due to musculoskeletal (MSK) disorders. Best Pract Res Clin Rheumatol 2014;28:353–366
14. Medical Expenditures Panel Survey [MEPS], Agency for Healthcare Research and Quality, U.S. Department of Health and Human Services, 2008–2011. Accessed at www.boneandjointburden.org/2014-report/xf3/medical-care-expenditures-and-earnings-losses-select-musculoskeletal-diseases; http://meps.ahrq.gov/mepsweb/
15. Murray CJ, Vos T, Lozano R, Naghavi M, Flaxman AD, Michaud C, Ezzati M, Shibuya K, Salomon JA, Abdalla S, et al. Disability-adjusted life years (DALYs) for 291 diseases and injuries in 21 regions, 1990–2010: a systematic analysis for the Global Burden of Disease Study 2010. Lancet 2012;380:2197–223.
16. National Health and Nutrition Examination Survey Questionnaire: NHANES 2003–2004. Accessed October 30, 2015 at http://cdcgov/nchs/nhanes/nhanes2003-2004/nhanes03_04htm.
17. Neogi T, Jansen TL, Dalbeth N, Fransen J, Schumacher HR, Berendsen D, Brown M, Choi H, Edwards NL, Janssens HJ, et al. 2015 Gout Classification Criteria: an American College of Rheumatology/European League Against Rheumatism collaborative initiative. Arthritis Rheum 2015;67:2557–68.
18. Nguyen UDT, Zhang Y, Niu J, Zhang B, Felson DT. Increasing prevalence of knee pain and symptomatic knee osteoarthritis. Arthritis Rheum 2010;62:S286.
19. Pleis JR, Lucas JW. Summary health statistics for U.S. adults: National Health Interview Survey, 2007. National Center for Health Statistics. Vital Health Stat 2009;10. Accessed at http://www.cdc.gov/nchs/data/series/sr_10/sr10_240.pdf
20. Sacks JJ, Helmick CG, Luo YH, Ilowite NT, Bowyer S. Prevalence of and annual ambulatory health care visits for pediatric arthritis and other rheumatologic conditions in the United States in 2001–2004. Arthritis Rheum 2007;57:1439–45.
21. Schiller JS, Lucas JW, Ward BW, Peregoy JA. Summary health statistics for U.S. adults: National Health Interview Survey, 2010. National Center for Health Statistics. Vital Health Stat 2012;10:1–207.
22. Vos T, Flaxman AD, Naghavi M, Lozano R, Michaud C, Ezzati M, Shibuya K, Salomon JA, Abdalla S, Aboyans V, et al. Years lived with disability (YLDs) for 1160 sequelae of 289 diseases and injuries 1990–2010: a systematic analysis for the Global Burden of Disease Study 2010. Lancet 2012;380:2163–96.
23. Yelin E, Murphy L, Cisternas MG, Foreman AJ, Pasta DJ, Helmick CG. Medical care expenditures and earnings losses among persons with arthritis and other rheumatic conditions in 2003, and comparisons with 1997. Arthritis Rheum 2007;56:1397–407.

CHAPTER 2

# Joint Neurophysiology and Pathophysiology (Nerves, Receptive Fields, Sensitization)

*Hans-Georg Schaible*

Joint pain is among the most frequent pain syndromes [3]. Reasons are manifold. Joints are often stressed by exhaustive physical challenges throughout life. They are a frequent site of injuries and degenerative processes during aging. Joints are preferential sites of inflammatory diseases due to metabolic disorders such as gout and autoimmune diseases (e.g., rheumatoid arthritis). Furthermore, the nociceptive system of muscle and joint is particularly prone to sensitization. This chapter addresses the nociceptive system of the joint, and it summarizes major changes in the nociceptive system during diseases of the joint.

## THE NOCICEPTIVE SYSTEM OF THE JOINT

### Nerve Supply of the Joint

The joint is supplied by thick myelinated Aβ fibers with corpuscular sensory endings (Ruffini-, Golgi-, Pacini-type) in ligaments, menisci, and fibrous joint capsule, and by sensory thin myelinated A∂ and unmyelinated C fibers with free sensory endings. The latter are located in all structures except the cartilage which is not innervated. In addition, joint nerves contain unmyelinated postganglionic sympathetic fibers [16].

## Response Properties of Aβ, A∂, and C Fibers of the Normal Joint

The sensory fibers have small receptive fields in the joint, that is, areas at which local stimulation with a mechanical probe elicits action potentials. Furthermore, many of them are activated by movements of the joint. According to their responsiveness to mechanical stimuli, sensory fibers are functionally characterized.

Aβ fibers with corpuscular sensory endings are proprioceptive. They have a low excitation threshold and show strong responses to innocuous mechanical stimuli such as movements in the working range and palpation of the joint. Their discharge rates may increase when noxious mechanical stimuli are applied to the joint. Noxious stimuli are movements beyond the working range against the resistance of the tissue, and strong pressure. However, Aβ fibers usually do not unequivocally encode noxious stimuli by their firing frequency, and they are not sensitized by chemical stimuli. Therefore, they are not considered nociceptors. They may sense the swelling of the inflamed joint.

About half of the A∂ fibers are also low-threshold fibers responding strongly to innocuous mechanical stimuli applied to the joint. However, the other A∂ fibers and most of the C fibers are nociceptive fibers because they preferentially or exclusively encode noxious mechanical stimuli applied to the joint. In line with the specificity theory of nociception, *specific nociceptive fibers* do respond only to stimuli of noxious intensity. A specific joint nociceptor does not respond to innocuous movements in the working range and to light or moderate pressure applied to the joint, but it responds to noxious (painful) stimuli such as rotation against the resistance of the tissue or strong pressure applied to the joint (hitting the joint). A typical joint nociceptor (C fiber) is displayed in Fig. 2-1 (left side). It has a small receptive field in the joint capsule (dot) with a high local mechanical excitation threshold; it does

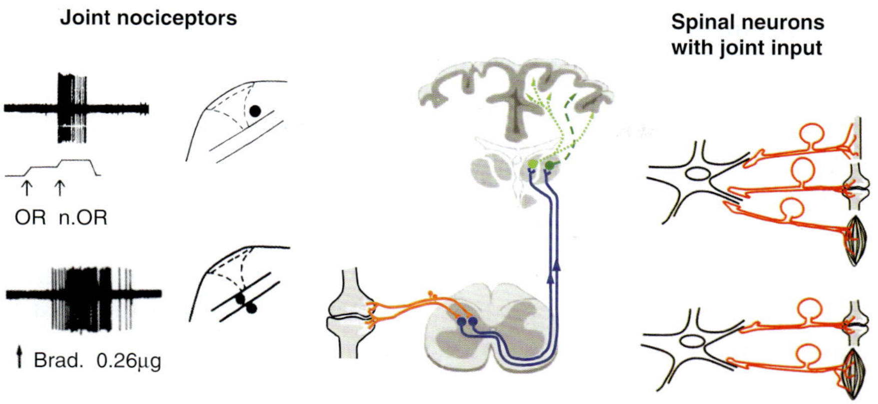


**FIGURE 2-1** Response properties of joint nociceptors **(left side)** and pattern of convergent inputs only from deep tissue or from deep tissue and the skin to spinal cord neurons with input from the joint **(right side)**. The panels on the left show action potentials elicited in joint nociceptors by noxious outward rotation (n.OR, supination) in the knee and by bradykinin. The spinal cord neurons, shown on the right side, receive either input from skin, joint, and muscle **(top)** or from deep tissue only **(bottom)**.

not respond to innocuous movements such as outward rotation (OR) but responds to noxious outward rotation (n.OR) against resistance.

Some A∂ and C fibers are weakly activated by movements in the working range and light pressure, but they show much stronger responses to noxious mechanical stimuli. Such neurons appear as wide-dynamic-range (WDR) neurons that encode innocuous and noxious stimulus intensities by their discharge rates. In addition, a proportion of sensory C fibers are silent nociceptors not responding to any innocuous and noxious mechanical stimulus applied to the normal joint [16].

Most of the A∂ and C fibers of the joint (both with low and high mechanical thresholds) respond to mechanical as well as to chemical stimuli. The chemosensitivity has several purposes. Some mediators directly excite the fibers at a short latency. In this way, noxious chemical stimuli may evoke pain. Such stimuli are hypertonic saline (4–6% NaCl), bradykinin (see typical response of a C fiber in Fig. 2-1, left side, bottom), serotonin, adenosine triphosphate (ATP), anandamide, adenosine receptor agonists, capsaicin, substance P, vasoactive intestinal peptide, galanin, and others (for review see [19]). The excitation is weak to strong and usually of short duration (in the range of seconds). A second purpose of chemosensitivity is the sensitization of the sensory fibers for mechanical stimuli. This function is particularly important in the context of inflammation in which allodynia and hyperalgesia are typical (see below). Sensitizing actions of mediators may be short lasting in the range of minutes (e.g., by bradykinin) or long lasting for hours up to days (e.g., by some proinflammatory cytokines and nerve growth factor [NGF], see below).

A model of the sensory ending of a nociceptor is displayed in Fig. 2-2. The membrane at the bottom side shows ion channels for the transduction of stimuli and voltage-activated ion channels for the generation of

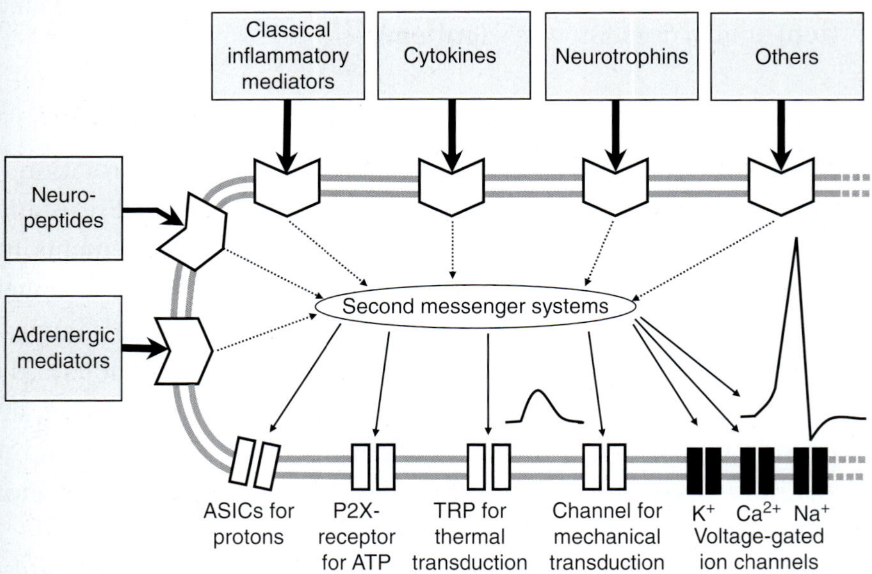


**FIGURE 2-2** Schematic drawing of a sensory ending of a nociceptor in the tissue. The membrane at the bottom shows ion channels for transduction (which produce a sensor potential), a voltage-gated $Na^+$ channel for the generation of action potentials (APs), and voltage-gated $K^+$ and $Ca^{2+}$ channels that control excitability. The other part of the membrane displays receptors for mediators that act on different second messenger systems. Classical inflammatory mediators are bradykinin, prostaglandin $E_2$, 5-hydroxytryptamine, and histamine. ASIC, acid-sensing ion channel; P2X, purinergic ion channel; TRP, transient receptor potential. (From Schaible et al. [18].)

action potentials and the control of neuronal excitability. The molecular structure of the channel(s) for the transduction of mechanical stimuli has not been identified. The sensory ending of a proportion of joint nociceptors expresses the transient receptor potential V1 (TRPV1) ion channel (usually activated by noxious heat), but the thermal sensitivity of joint afferents has not been explored. The chemosensitivity either rests on ion channels, which are opened by mediators (e.g., acid-sensing ion channels [ASICs] by protons, P2X channels by ATP, TRPV1 channels by capsaicin), or is produced by metabotropic receptors in the membrane that bind the mediator and activate second messenger system which then open ion channels (Fig. 2-2, membrane at the top side). Such receptors are B receptors for bradykinin, P2Y receptors for ATP, EP receptors for $PGE_2$, and many others. In addition to excitatory and/or sensitizing mediators, mediators with inhibitory functions may also act on neuronal receptors (e.g., opioids, somatostatin) [16, 20].

## Spinal Cord Neurons That Process Nociceptive Sensory Input from the Joint

Uptake of horseradish peroxidase by joint nerves was used to visualize the projection of the joint nerves into the spinal cord. Sensory fibers of the joint project to the superficial dorsal horn and to the deep dorsal horn. Whether the spinal projections of A and C fibers from the joint differ has not been investigated. Typically, primary sensory neurons from a joint project into several segments. Electrophysiologically, spinal cord neurons with input from the joint are identified in the superficial and deep dorsal horn [16].

In the rat, a typical spinal cord neuron with input from the knee joint shows receptive fields in the knee joint, in the adjacent muscles of thigh and lower leg, and in the ankle joint. Even the paw may be included in the receptive field. Such neurons are either excited only from deep tissue or show in addition receptive fields in the skin (Fig. 2-1, right side). Often, the cutaneous receptive field is located more distally than the receptive fields in deep tissue, thus allowing separate stimulation of skin and deep tissue. Many neurons with deep input only have high thresholds and are activated only by noxious stimuli applied to the joint and muscles as long as the joint is healthy. Most of the neurons with additional cutaneous receptive fields are WDR neurons. Upon stimulation of the joint, they have activation thresholds in the innocuous range but encode a whole range of innocuous and noxious intensities by their discharge frequencies [16]. Neurons with input from the joint project to supraspinal sites (cerebellum, spinocervical nucleus, thalamus, reticular formation) or to intraspinal (segmental) interneurons and motoneurons [16].

Most spinal cord neurons with joint and muscle input are tonically inhibited by descending inhibitory systems, which originate in the brain stem and modulate spinal cord activity. The interruption of descending inhibition lowers their excitation threshold for mechanical stimulation, substantially increases their responses to suprathreshold stimulation and the size of their receptive fields, and causes (increased) ongoing discharges. Neurons with joint input are also inhibited by heterotopic noxious stimuli, in line with the concept of diffuse noxious inhibitory control (DNIC), thus implying that painful stimulation at one site of the body may reduce the pain at another site of the body [16].

## Processing of Nociceptive Input from the Joint in the Brain

Ascending spinal cord neurons with joint input activate the cortical pain matrix, thus evoking the conscious pain sensation. The medial system of the pain matrix (anterior cingulate cortex, insula, and thalamus) is particularly activated [9]. Differences between the processing of cutaneous and deep input have not been clearly worked out yet.

In the thalamus, WDR neurons with convergent cutaneous and deep input were found in the ventral and dorsolateral periphery of the ventroposterolateral nucleus (VPL) and in the transitional zone between VPL and the ventrolateral nucleus. In the rat, nociceptive neurons with input from skin and joints were intermingled with tactile neurons throughout the ventrobasal complex. In cats, nociceptive neurons with very large and often bilateral receptive fields and convergent inputs from skin and deep tissue were identified in the posterior complex and in the medial nucleus of the thalamus. The somatosensory cortex in rats contains a large proportion of neurons that respond to noxious stimulation, and a small proportion of these neurons is driven by deep input. Electrical stimulation of Aβ and A∂ fibers in the posterior articular nerve of rat's knee evoked field potentials in cortical SI and SII [16].

Neurons with convergent inputs from skin and deep tissue including the joint also activate the amygdala. The latter are thought to provide emotional-affective modulation of cognitive functions in pain; they may contribute to the integration of pain, fear, and anxiety; and they show connections to the cortex as well as to the periaqueductal gray (PAG), the region in the brain stem from which the descending inhibitory systems originate [13].

## NEURONAL CHANGES EVOKED BY INFLAMMATION IN THE JOINT

Diseases of the joint are typically characterized by inflammatory components, and in the course of such diseases, the joint develops allodynia and hyperalgesia. Allodynia manifests itself as pain experienced during movements in the working range of the joint and pain upon palpation, hyperalgesia as strong pain upon noxious stimulation. Because of these features, joint pain is typically considered nociceptive. However, even in inflammatory models, a neuropathic component may develop in the course of disease, which may be manifest after the remission of the inflammatory phase [4].

Inflammation-evoked changes are elicited at all levels of the neuraxis. The relative importance of mechanisms at the different levels may determine the pain pattern in individual patients [5, 15]. Such changes are the peripheral sensitization, the central sensitization (in particular spinal sensitization), changes in the pain matrix, and changes in descending inhibitory systems (Fig. 2-3).

### Peripheral Sensitization

During pathological changes in the joint, polymodal joint nociceptors are particularly sensitized for mechanical stimuli. This is a significant

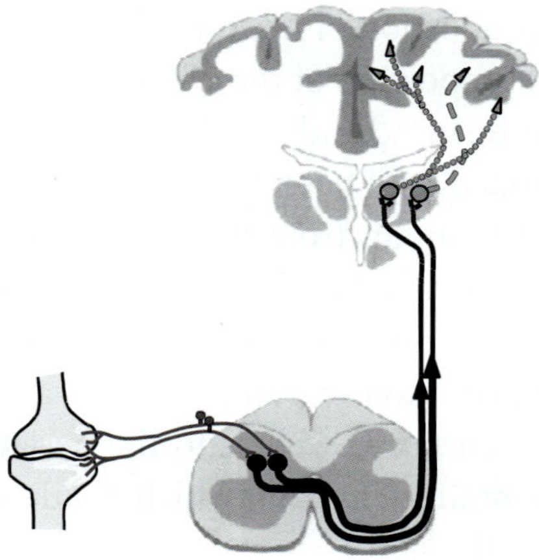


**FIGURE 2-3** Overview of changes in the nociceptive system of the joint during chronic joint diseases.

difference to cutaneous nociceptors which are particularly sensitized to heat stimuli. Mechanical sensitization is characterized by the lowering of the excitation threshold from the noxious range to the innocuous range and an increase of responses to noxious stimuli. Thus, the nociceptor, displayed in Fig. 2-1, will develop strong responses to OR and other movements in the working range. Sensitization may also be observed in non-nociceptive polymodal sensory fibers. In addition, silent nociceptors are sensitized and become responsive to mechanical stimuli. The recruitment of silent fibers increases the peripheral input into the spinal cord [16].

## Molecular Mechanisms of Peripheral Mechanical Sensitization

As mentioned above, some mediators that excite neurons may also (transiently) increase the mechanosensitivity of the polymodal neurons, by activating second messenger systems that alter the opening characteristics of the ion channels (Fig. 2-2). Such actions were reported for $PGE_2$, $PGI_2$, bradykinin, glutamate, ATP, 5-HT, protons, and others [19]. Of particular interest are mediators that induce sensitization lasting for hours or days. Such effects are mainly attributed to growth factors and proinflammatory cytokines. Long-lasting sensitization may also be induced by mediators that activate protease-activated receptors [11].

In the joint, NGF plays a role because it enhances osteoarthritic pain [2]. A single injection of an antibody to NGF improved osteoarthritis (OA) pain in humans for several weeks [10]. In joint nociception also the effect of proinflammatory cytokines was studied because these mediators are central to rheumatology. Tumor necrosis factor (TNF), IL-6, IL-1β, and IL-17 induce at a slow time course, a state of long-lasting mechanical sensitization of nociceptive C fibers of the joint. TNF also sensitizes A∂ fibers. Interestingly, IL-1β and IL-17 at low doses rather desensitize A∂ fibers. Neutralization of proinflammatory cytokines can reduce mechanical sensitization and mechanical hyperalgesia in human rheumatoid arthritis and experimental models of rheumatoid arthritis [17].

The long-lasting mechanical sensitization is due to an increase of the sensitivity of ion channels (e.g., sodium channels), and some findings suggest that TRP channels such as TRPA1 and TRPV4 are also involved. The contribution of TRPV1 was also proposed [17, 18].

### Reduction of Mechanical Hyperexcitability

Sensory endings also express receptors for inhibitory mediators. Opioids and somatostatin reduce the enhanced inflammation-evoked activity [20]. The TRPV1 receptor agonist capsaicin desensitizes nociceptors for mechanical stimuli [18]. Interestingly, even the EP3 receptor for $PGE_2$ reduces inflammation-evoked mechanical sensitization upon inflammation [12].

## Spinal Sensitization

In the course of joint inflammation, spinal cord neurons with joint input develop a state of hyperexcitability. In high-threshold spinal neurons, the threshold is lowered into the innocuous range such that they respond to innocuous stimuli. In all nociceptive neurons, the responses to noxious stimuli increase. These increases are observed not only for stimuli applied to the inflamed region, but also for stimuli applied to adjacent and remote areas. In addition, the whole receptive field of the neuron can show considerable expansion (Fig. 2-4). Because of the development of hyperexcitability and the expansion of the receptive fields of neurons, the population of neurons responding to stimulation expands in the segments with input from inflamed deep tissue. These spinal changes explain the occurrence of areas of primary hyperalgesia (at the site of inflammation) and secondary hyperalgesia (in areas remote from the inflamed area) [16]. Central sensitization can persist during chronic inflammation or even outlast peripheral mechanisms [15]. The spinal sensitization is thought to correspond to the expansion of the hyperalgesic areas in the leg in humans upon noxious stimulation, a typical phenomenon in patients with local joint diseases [1]. Patients with chronic pain in a joint may even develop widespread pain [15].

Spinal sensitization is influenced by pathways from the brain stem. At the acute stage of inflammation, tonic descending inhibition as well as heterotopic inhibitory influences are increased, but this is not sustained at the chronic stage of inflammation [16]. In patients, the inhibition by heterotopic influences (DNIC) is actually reduced during severe OA but is restored after replacement of the osteoarthritic hip joint [8]. Thus, elementary descending endogenous pain control systems may

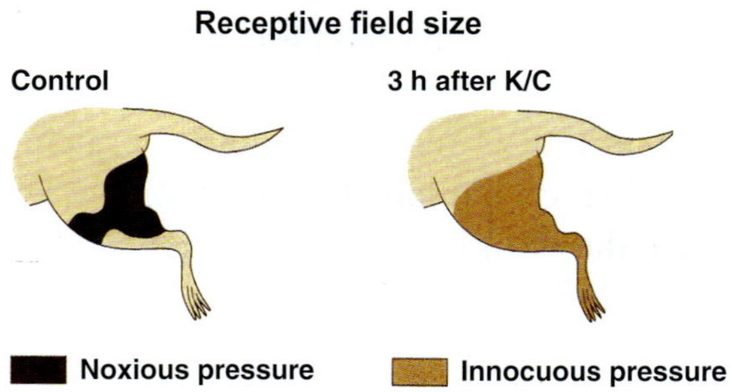


**FIGURE 2-4** Expansion of the receptive field of a spinal cord neuron with joint input by inflammation in the knee. Before inflammation, the neuron had a high mechanical excitation threshold in the knee and adjacent muscles **(black area)**; at 3 hours after induction of joint inflammation by kaolin/carrageenan (K/C), the receptive field was expanded in thigh and to the paw, and the local mechanical threshold for excitation dropped into the innocuous range (excitation by palpation).

actually be insufficient under chronic pain conditions in OA and rheumatoid arthritis [1].

### Molecular Mechanisms

The generation and maintenance of central sensitization is produced by the action of transmitter/receptor systems in the spinal cord. After sensitization, primary afferent neurons release more transmitters from their spinal terminations upon peripheral stimulation (presynaptic component). Furthermore, spinal cord neurons are rendered more excitable by changes in receptor sensitivity (postsynaptic component). In addition, spinal glia activation (astrocyte and microglia) may contribute to the sensitization process [14].

Glutamate plays a key role because it activates *N*-methyl-D-aspartate (NMDA) receptors upon noxious stimuli applied to deep tissue. The activation of NMDA receptors is critically involved in the generation and maintenance of spinal hyperexcitability. The spinal sensitization is facilitated by neuropeptides such as substance P and calcitonin gene-related peptide (CGRP). It is also furthered by spinal prostaglandins (in particular by $PGE_2$) which are produced by an upregulation of spinal cyclooxygenases. However, the presence of spinal $PGE_2$ seems to be required for the generation but not for the maintenance of spinal hyperexcitability [16]. But the role of spinal PGs is more complex. $PGD_2$, another major PG in the central nervous system, dose-dependently reduced responses of spinal cord neurons to stimulation of the inflamed knee joint, whereas an antagonist at the DP1 receptor increased responses [16]. Indeed, $PGD_2$ counteracts the sensitizing effects of $PGE_2$, in line with the view that $PGD_2$ is neuroprotective in the brain, via DP1 receptors. Spinal sensitization during joint inflammation is also supported by spinal cytokines (e.g., spinal TNF and spinal IL-6) [7]. Spinal hyperexcitability may be counteracted by endocannabinoids and other inhibitory receptors [16].

## Changes in the Brain

Considerable changes of the processing of deep input were observed at inflammatory states. In polyarthritic rats, a large proportion of neurons in the ventrobasal complex of the thalamus respond to movements and gentle pressure onto inflamed joints (often with long lasting after discharges), whereas only few neurons respond to these stimuli in normal rats. Some neurons also displayed paroxysmal discharges. Furthermore, neurons in the nucleus centralis lateralis acquire input from the inflamed joint, which is not present in normal animals. Similarly, neurons in superficial cortical layers do not respond to joint stimulation in normal rats but start to respond to joint stimulation in polyarthritic rats. These findings indicate substantial neuroplasticity at the thalamocortical level that may contribute to inflammatory deep tissue pain [16].

Brain imaging in patients with pain in the joint shows an activation of the pain matrix [9]. On the other hand, chronic OA patients exhibited signs of atrophy in thalamus and the gray matter of pain-related cortical areas, but these were reversible after arthroplasty [6].

## EFFERENT EFFECTS OF THE NERVOUS SYSTEM ON THE JOINT

The innervation of joints has not only sensory functions. The nervous system can also influence the milieu of the joint and modify inflammation. The neuronal pathways for efferent functions are the following:

**a.** Upon activation, peptidergic nociceptive sensory C fibers of the joint release neuropeptides such as CGRP and substance P in the tissue, and these neuropeptides can produce neurogenic inflammation.

**b.** Postganglionic fibers of the sympathetic nervous system continuously control the blood flow in the joint. The sympathetic nervous system can further inflammation but in some experimental models also inhibit inflammatory changes at advanced stages of inflammation.

**c.** The spinal cord can support inflammation by the generation of dorsal root reflexes (retrograde activity in nociceptive fibers and release of neuropeptides in the joint) and via the sympathetic nervous system. Thus, central sensitization is not only involved in pain generation.

d. Neuroendocrine systems such as the hypothalamic–pituitary–adrenal axis can modify inflammation [16].

Together with the immune system, the nervous system determines the inflammatory process.

## REFERENCES

1. Arendt-Nielsen L, Eskehave TN, Egsgaard LL, Petersen KK, Graven-Nielsen T, Hoeck HC, Simonsen O, Siebuhr AS, Karsdal M, Bay-Jensen AC. Association between experimental pain biomarkers and serologic markers in patients with different degrees of painful knee osteoarthritis. Arthritis Rheum 2014;66:3317–26.
2. Ashraf S, Mapp PI, Burston J, Bennett AJ, Chapman V, Walsh DA. Augmented pain behavioural responses to intra-articular injection of growth factor in two animal models of osteoarthritis. Ann Rheum Dis 2014;73:1710–18.
3. Breivik H, Collet B, Ventafridda V, Cohen R, Gallacher D. Survey of chronic pain in Europe. Eur J Pain 2006;10:287–333.
4. Christianson CA, Corr M, Firestein GS, Mobargha A, Yaksh TL, Svensson C. Characterization of the acute and persistent pain state present in K/BxN serum transfer arthritis. Pain 2010;151:394–403.
5. Egsgaard LL, Eskehave TN, Bay-Jensen AC, Hoeck HC, Arendt-Nielsen L. Identifying specific profiles in patients with different degrees of painful knee osteoarthritis based on serological biochemical and mechanistic pain biomarkers: a diagnostic approach based on cluster analysis. Pain 2015;156:96–107.
6. Gwilym SE, Filippini N, Douaud G, Carr AJ, Tracey I. Thalamic atrophy associated with painful osteoarthritis of the hip is reversible after arthroplasty. Arthritis Rheum 2010;62:2930–40.
7. König C, Zharsky M, Möller C, Schaible H-G, Ebersberger A. Involvement of peripheral and spinal tumor-necrosis-factor (TNF) in spinal cord hyperexcitability during knee joint inflammation in rat. Arthritis Rheum 2014;66:599–609.
8. Kosek E, Ordeberg G. Lack of pressure pain modulation by heterotopic noxious conditioning stimulation in patients with painful osteoarthritis before, but not following surgical pain relief. Pain 2000;88:69–78.
9. Kulkarni B, Bentley DE, Elliott R, Julyan PJ, Boger E, Watson A, Boyle Y, El-Deredy W, Jones AK. Arthritic pain is processed in brain areas concerned with emotions and fear. Arthritis Rheum 2007;56:1345–54.
10. Lane NE, Schnitzer TJ, Birbara CA, Mokhtarani M, Shelton DL, Smith MD, Brown MT. Tanezumab for the treatment of pain from osteoarthritis of the knee. N Engl J Med 2010;363:1521–31.
11. McDougall JJ, Muley MM. The role of proteases in pain. In: Schaible H-G, editor. Pain control. Berlin: Springer; 2015. p. 239–60.
12. Natura G, Bär K-J, Eitner A, Böttger M, Richter F, Hensellek S, Ebersberger A, Leuchtweis J, Maruyama T, Hofmann GO, et al. Neuronal prostaglandin E2

receptor subtype EP3 mediates antinociception during inflammation. Proc Natl Acad Sci USA 2013;110:13648–53.
13. Neugebauer V, Li W, Bird GC, Han JS. The amygdala and persistent pain. Neuroscientist 2004;10:221–34.
14. Ogbonna AC, Clark AK, Gentry C, Hobbs C, Malcangio M. Pain-like behavior and spinal changes in the monosodium iodoacetate model of osteoarthritis in C57Bl/6 mice. Eur J Pain 2013;17:514–26.
15. Phillips K, Clauw DJ. Central pain mechanisms in the rheumatic diseases. Arthritis Rheum 2013;65:291–302.
16. Schaible H-G. Joint pain: basic mechanisms. In: McMahon SB, Tracey I, Koltzenburg M, Turk DC, editors. Wall and Melzack's textbook of pain, 6th edition. Philadelphia: Elsevier Saunders; 2013. p. 609–19.
17. Schaible H-G. Nociceptive neurons detect cytokines in arthritis. Arthritis Res Ther 2014;16:470.
18. Schaible H-G, Ebersberger A, Natura G. Update on peripheral mechanisms of pain: beyond prostaglandins and cytokines. Arthritis Res Ther 2011;13:210.
19. Schaible H-G, Richter F. Receptors relevant for joint nociception. In: Graven-Nielsen T, Arendt-Nielsen L, editors. Musculoskeletal pain: basic mechanisms and implications. Washington DC: IASP Press; 2014. p. 187–204.
20. Stein C, Clark JD, Oh U, Vasko MR, Wilcox GL, Overland AC, Vanderah TW, Spencer RH. Peripheral mechanisms of pain and analgesia. Brain Res Rev 2009;60:90–113.

CHAPTER 3

# Animal Models of Osteoarthritic Pain

*Devi Rani Sagar, Sadaf Ashraf, and Victoria Chapman*

Osteoarthritis (OA) is the fastest growing chronic pain disease worldwide [37, 63] and is the most common form of arthritis, with the prevalence of OA increasing with age [17]. OA is a heterogeneous multifactorial disorder with genetic and environmental risk factors accelerating its progression. Psychological factors such as low mood and anxiety can also augment OA pain and modify the pain experience. All compartments of OA joints undergo structural changes, impairing function, causing disability, and reducing quality of life [17]. Recent clinical and preclinical evidence supports bidirectional interactions between cartilage and subchondral bone turnover in OA, and the contribution of subchondral bone mechanisms to the pathogenesis, pain, and progression of OA is increasingly evident [26]. Articular cartilage and the adjacent subchondral bone plate protect the subchondral bone, both biomechanically and from biochemical influences from the synovial cavity. The importance of this barrier function is evident from the efficacy of total joint replacement, which replaces articular cartilage with a noncompressible and impermeable prosthesis, protecting subchondral bone and substantially relieving pain for most of the patients. However, increasing demand led to >92,000 primary knee replacements in England in 2012/2013, costing approximately £500 million per year [12].

The challenge of identification of effective analgesic strategies for OA pain arises in part because of the heterogeneity of the disease and the pain associated with it. It is widely acknowledged that the severity of OA with respect to histopathological changes does not always correlate with extent of OA pain experienced [20]. Pain perception and processing differs greatly between people at different stages of the disease. OA pain is experienced while resting, on weight-bearing, or on joint movement. A proportion of patients experience pain in areas outside of the joint indicative of central sensitization [3]. The complexity of OA pain means that treatments targeting one specific mechanism may have low efficacy if offered to people whose pain is largely mediated by other mechanisms. Treatment guidelines, therefore, recommend that the optimal management of OA should be tailored according to patient characteristics, including pain phenotyping [68]. Quantitative sensory testing (QST) is one approach for mechanism-based phenotyping of OA pain [43]. Pain responses can be assessed at the affected site or at a remote site to the diseased joint. Localized pain at the affected joint is associated with peripheral sensitization, whereas pain at a site adjacent to, or at a distance from, the site of origin suggests a combination of peripheral and central sensitization. A recently conducted systematic review of the use of QST to characterize pain in people with OA, compared with controls, demonstrated that people with OA had lower pressure pain thresholds (PPTs) both at the affected joint and at remote sites not directly affected by OA, indicating a contribution of central sensitization mechanisms [56].

Synovitis and subchondral bone marrow lesions (BMLs) are most commonly associated with OA pain. Magnetic resonance imaging (MRI), increasingly used to evaluate joint pathology in OA, plays a critical role in the visualization of pathological and structural changes, including BMLs, which cannot be seen on conventional radiographs [20]. BMLs are noncystic subchondral areas of ill-defined high signal intensity directly adjacent to cartilage on T2-weighted, fat-saturated, or short tau inversion recovery (STIR) images on MRI. BMLs in knee OA are associated with pain, in both cross-sectional and longitudinal studies [13].

Not only are current analgesics poorly effective at treating OA pain, but they can also have numerous adverse effects. The lack of an effective treatment protocol to control OA pain and progression represents an enormous unmet medical need and underpins the necessity to better understand the pathophysiology of OA. Paracetamol and/or topical nonsteroidal anti-inflammatory drugs (NSAIDS) are the recommended first-line analgesic agents in OA, and oral NSAIDS or cyclooxygenase-2 (COX-2) inhibitors are used when these are inadequate [38]. Novel pharmacological targets which sequester nerve growth factor (NGF) have good efficacy in preclinical and clinical studies in improving OA pain, but are not yet used routinely in clinics [30].

Reducing pain, increasing joint function, and halting disease progression are the three main goals for new improved OA therapies. To develop such therapies, an in-depth understanding of the pathophysiology of OA is required, using both relevant animal models that best mimic disease progression and OA pain and clinical samples where available. Currently used animal models of OA illustrate the challenge in modeling the complexity of OA pain; no one model replicates OA in humans, but each model can be used to study specific aspects of the disease, which may, in turn, have translational validity for different clinical subgroups. In this chapter, we review the most widely studied rodent models of OA pain and discuss the various strengths and weaknesses of these models in mimicking aspects of human OA pain and their translational validity. While OA is a disease which may affect many different types of joint, for the purposes of this chapter, we will focus on models of knee OA.

## ANIMAL MODELS

Until recently, structural changes within the joint have been the main focus of preclinical OA studies. Since pain is the most important and debilitating feature of OA, in vivo studies are also focusing on elucidating OA pain mechanisms using various models and methods of assessment (Tables 3-1 and 3-2). Animals that spontaneously develop OA (including genetically modified animals) [57] appear to offer the most translatable and relevant models of OA; however, the development of spontaneous

**TABLE 3-1 A Comparison of Commonly Used Measures of Knee Pain Employed in Animal Models of OA**

| Measures of Knee Pain | Test Methods | Outcome Measures | Animal Models |
|---|---|---|---|
| Compression of knee joint | Pressing knee joint either manually or using a computerized calibrated forceps | Vocalization, struggle, withdrawal | Chemical<br>Inflammatory |
| Struggle threshold angle of knee extension/flexion | Tibia is extended while femur is held in position | Vocalization, struggle | Chemical<br>Inflammatory |
| Static weight-bearing | Incapacitance | Hind limb weight distribution as the force exerted by each limb on a transducer plate over a given period of time. | Chemical<br>Inflammatory<br>Surgical |
| Posture and gait analysis | Stationary or dynamic<br>Forced exercise<br>Forced ambulation | Behavioral signs, limping, curling toes, guarding, speed, avoiding contact with limb. | Chemical<br>Inflammatory<br>Surgical |
| Mechanical or heat sensitivity of the paw | Von Frey/Randall Selitto<br>Heat source<br>Cooling effect | Withdrawal threshold or latency. Vocalization, struggle. Behavioral signs, flinching, shaking, toe biting. | Chemical<br>Inflammatory<br>Surgical |
| Grip strength | Grip strength | Maximum force displayed by an animal | Chemical |

OA by its very nature can be unpredictable and occur over a long period of time, which presents challenges for studying the mechanisms underpinning the pathogenesis of OA. Experimenter-induced OA models (inflammatory, chemical, surgical, and genetically modified) provide an opportunity to investigate the mechanisms of pain related to specific pathological changes at different time points in the progression of OA.

## ASSESSING PAIN IN ANIMAL MODELS

Many different measures are used to evaluate nociceptive responses in models of OA (Table 3-1). Common measures include changes in

TABLE 3-2 **Key Features of Commonly Used Animal Models of OA Pain and Use in Combination with Genetically Modified Mice**

| Animal Models of OA Pain | Key Features | Combined with Genetically Modified Mice | Pain Assessment |
|---|---|---|---|
| Spontaneous | Clinically relevant. High variability of disease phenotype and incidence. Timely. Large experimental groups. Difficulty in obtaining age-matched controls. | N/A | N/A |
| Inflammatory | Represents one feature of OA pathology. Acute and chronic. | N/A | N/A |
| Surgical | Can be controlled to model rapid and severe onset of OA or slow and mild disease progression. Injury has clinical relevance. | ADAMTS-5 and GDF-5 | Yes [11, 32] |
| Chemical | Can be controlled to model rapid and severe onset of OA, or mild disease. Robust reproducible pain model. No need for sham control. | N/A | N/A |
| Genetically modified | Offers potential to understand molecular mechanisms of OA initiation and progression. Can be used as a background for experimenter-induced OA. Sex, age, and background need appropriate controls; need to verify pathogen status. | Type IX collagen | Yes [2] |

N/A, no available data.

weight distribution between the injured and uninjured hind limb. This can be achieved in a number of ways; incapacitance testing is a measure of static weight-bearing, whereas gait analysis and dynamic weight-bearing can identify changes in weight distribution on movement. These measures are reproducible in terms of nociceptive responses in models of OA; however, their sensitivity depends on the severity of OA. Changes in weight distribution can be used only in models of unilateral injury and so cannot be used in spontaneously occurring models of OA pain. Hind limb grip strength is also measured in models of OA and may represent a more sensitive measure of analgesic efficacy in models of OA [23, 24]. Systematic review of the different methods to assess pain in animal models of OA and the prediction of the efficacy of drugs to reduce OA pain responses concluded that grip strength was the most sensitive measure of OA pain [55]. Thermally and mechanically evoked pain tests are used to measure hyperalgesia and allodynia, respectively. These include hind limb paw withdrawal thresholds measured in response to increased pressure stimuli (Von Frey filaments) applied to the plantar surface and thermal sensitivity of the paw measured using the hot-plate test to measure paw withdrawal latency. Alterations in mechanical withdrawal thresholds at distal sites, such as the hind paw, are often used to demonstrate the presence of alterations in nociceptive processing in areas outside the joint. Other tests used include the measurement of reflexes and/or knee-compression-evoked vocalization [16], reduced range of motion, and mechanical sensitivity of the knee by measuring the struggle threshold [51].

## SPONTANEOUS MODELS

Naturally occurring OA models probably mimic the causes, histopathological features, and slow rates of progression of human disease better than the experimenter-induced models. Dunkin Hartley Guinea pigs, and some strains of mice (STR/ort, C57Black), spontaneously develop OA joint pathology [44]. Most of the studies of spontaneous OA models have focused on the structural damage to the joints, as the assessment of pain responses in these models is challenging because the disease occurs bilaterally, which precludes changes in weight-bearing as an index of pain. As a result, other methods of quantifying pain responses have been employed, including the firing frequencies of afferent fibers innervating the joint. Electrophysiological studies in aged

Dunkin Hartley Guinea pigs reported increased spontaneous activity and enhanced neuronal firing to noxious joint movement, compared with younger Guinea pigs, both of which are indicative of peripheral sensitization of joint afferents [34]. This study did not find a significant correlation between severity of joint pathology and nociceptive responses in this model, which is consistent with findings from clinical studies.

A limitation of the spontaneous models is that, like the human condition, there is a high degree of variability in time of onset and the rate and extent of pathological progression between animals, which leads to a heterogeneous population and a need for larger experimental group sizes. In addition, it is not always possible to use an appropriate age-matched, nonarthritic control from which meaningful and ultimately translatable comparisons can be made. Since spontaneous models of OA develop slowly, they require long periods of housing, raising ethical and practical issues. Some of these concerns can be addressed by the use of experimenter-induced models of OA pain, discussed below.

## INFLAMMATORY MODELS

Recurrent inflammatory phases are common in human OA. Acute and chronic phases of inflammation can be modeled in animals through the injections of chemicals like kaolin/carrageenan (K/C). Intra-articular injections of kaolin/carrageenan into knee joints produce cartilage damage, synovitis, and synovial fluid exudates. K/C arthritis develops rapidly within hours and persists for weeks. Pathological, behavioral, and electrophysiological changes have been studied extensively in the K/C arthritis model [22, 39, 53, 67]. A modification of the K/C arthritis model is the injection of carrageenan alone, the time course of this type of arthritis is shorter (hours to days), and the cartilage damage is less pronounced [15, 36, 59]. Other models of knee inflammation include the chronic complete Freund's adjuvant (CFA)–induced arthritis by intra-articular injection of CFA [16, 35, 51, 54, 66]. CFA is characterized by joint inflammation, cartilage destruction, pannus and bone erosion, which can persist for at least a month. In these models of inflammatory arthritis, pain has been measured by assessment of gait [59], spontaneous mobility [19], paw withdrawal thresholds [52], mechanical sensitivity of the knee [16, 66], and measuring knee extension angle at which the animal displays a struggle response as an index of pain [51, 66]. Inflammation is a key component of OA, and therefore, these models can provide insight into the mechanisms of joint inflammation as a causative factor in OA pain.

## GENETICALLY MODIFIED MODELS

OA is known to have a significant genetic contribution [61]. Knockout or transgenic mice strains alone, or in combination with chemically/surgically induced OA, can provide an invaluable resource to examine genetic predispositions/contributions to OA as recently reviewed [62] (Table 3-2). Model standardization is crucial as genetic background, sex, and age of animals can significantly impact upon outcome measures, including pain behavioral responses. Appropriate controls are essential but become complex with conditional knockout mice and mixed strain backgrounds. Pathogen status of mice also needs to be evaluated as it can affect the incidence and severity of inflammatory arthritis. Most studies using knockout/transgenic mice models have focused on assessing the structural features of joint pathology rather than pain responses. Cre recombinase lines driven by cartilage-expressing molecules such as aggrecan, type II collagen, and growth/differentiation factor-5 (GDF-5) have been generated for studies of OA mechanisms [9, 47, 62]. In a recent study, mice deficient for a disintegrin and metalloproteinase with thrombospondin motifs 5 (ADAMTS-5), a key aggrecanase involved in accelerating OA and compromising joint integrity, did not develop pathology or pain behavior following induction of an established surgical model of OA [32]. Other pain modalities, including thermal hyperalgesia, locomotor activity, and gait analysis, did not show significant differences between groups. Type IX collagen deficient mice developed knee OA and exhibited compensatory gait changes, increased mechanical sensitivity, and impaired physical ability assessed by contact righting, wire hang, rotarod, and pole climbing [2]. These gait and functional differences suggest that type IX collagen deficient mice select locomotive behaviors that limit joint loads. The nature and magnitude of behavioral changes were largest in males, which also had the greatest evidence of knee OA.

## SURGICAL MODELS

Instability of the joint resulting from internal derangements of the joint has been shown to be a precipitating factor in the incidence of OA in humans; therefore, many models of OA use a surgical intervention in an attempt to replicate posttraumatic OA. Joint instability as a result of transection of anterior cruciate or medial collateral ligaments produces OA-like histopathological changes of the joint, which is accompanied by pain behavior [6]. Models involving transection of the meniscus (MNX) can replicate injuries such as meniscal tears, and lead to OA-like histopathology. From as early as 2 weeks following meniscal transection surgery, histopathological changes such as cartilage fibrillation, osteophyte formation, proteoglycan loss, and chondrocyte death can be seen, which progress with time [6, 7]. The MNX model is associated with the development of pain behavioral responses, specifically weight-bearing asymmetry and lowered hind paw withdrawal thresholds [5, 40]. All models of surgical OA exhibit early postoperative pain responses [5, 32] prior to the presence of structural OA. However, from around 2 weeks post-surgery, soft tissues have repaired and OA-like joint pathology, and associated pain behavior is evident and maintained for at least 7 weeks post-surgery [33]. The rapid onset of pathological changes and pain behavior in the MNX model do not allow for early events occurring in OA to be studied, which has led to the development of variations of the surgical interventions to produce less rapidly developing models. Destabilization of the medial meniscus (DMM) in mice has been demonstrated to be a slower progressing model compared with the MNX model, with distinct phases of pain behavior [25, 32] and gender differences [32]. This model exhibits significant differences in weight-bearing on the ipsilateral hind limb 12 weeks post-surgery compared with sham-operated mice [25], and, therefore, may be more useful for the evaluation of mechanisms associated with the early stages of OA pain.

There have been a limited number of studies of the impact of surgical models of OA on the nociceptive pathways. Electrophysiological recordings from dorsal root ganglion (DRG) neurons in vivo demonstrated that response properties of low-threshold mechanoreceptors, including muscle afferents, were altered following surgical derangement of the knee joint in rats [64, 65]. This change in function of non-nociceptive neurons in OA may reflect a phenotypic change capable of providing a novel input to the central pain pathways, which contributes to spinal plasticity in OA [64, 65]. Few studies have been done on the potential alterations in supraspinal activity in surgical models of OA. An imaging study demonstrated increased functional connectivity in the nucleus accumbens and ventral posterior lateral thalamus in MNX rats at 3 weeks post-surgery [60]. Further studies of the supraspinal changes associated with OA pain behavior using animal models will be invaluable.

## MONOSODIUM IODOACETATE MODEL

Chemical models of OA offer the advantage that they are minimally invasive and do not require the use of sham-operated controls; they have a rapid onset of action, and most models produce robust and reproducible pain behavior. Monosodium iodoacetate (MIA) is a metabolic inhibitor of chondrocyte glyceraldehyde-3-phosphate dehydrogenase, which disrupts glycolysis and results in cell death. Intra-articular injection of MIA produces rapid chondrocyte and proteoglycan loss [7], which is associated with dose-dependent histopathological changes. Depending on the concentration of MIA used, the extent of chondrocyte death can differ from that seen in human OA [44]. In both rats and mice, changes in weight-bearing and decreased paw withdrawal thresholds of the ipsilateral hind limbs are evident from as early as day 3 postinjection and are maintained for at least 9 weeks in rats [10] and 4 weeks in mice [41]. Two weeks following MIA injection, OA structural changes mimic human pathology [18, 33] and increased neuronal excitability within the peripheral nervous system is evident; specifically, C-fiber joint nociceptors had increased rates of spontaneous activity accompanied by decreased thresholds, and Aδ-fiber joint nociceptors had increased evoked firing rates [28]. Similarly at slightly later time points, hind-paw A- and C-fiber-evoked responses of spinal neurons are facilitated at 14–21 days in the MIA model in the mouse [21]. As well as changes to neuronal activity, elevations in pronociceptive neuropeptides substance P and calcitonin gene-related protein (CGRP) have been demonstrated in both the periphery [1] and the spinal cord [14]. Electrophysiological studies have shown that blockade of endogenous CGRP reversed MIA-induced enhancement of joint nociceptor responses [8]. Augmented stimulation-evoked release of CGRP from the spinal terminals of primary afferents has been demonstrated at 3–4 weeks after intra-articular injection of MIA in the mouse, compared to controls [41]. Collectively, these data indicate that changes in CGRP contribute to the peripheral and central sensitization exhibited in experimental OA. As with human OA, NGF has been demonstrated to have pronociceptive effects in vivo [4]. Intra-articular injection of NGF enhanced pain behavior in OA rats [4] and produced enhanced knee-extension-evoked firing of spinal neurons as well as an expansion of the peripheral receptive fields of neurons in MIA rats, compared with saline-injected rats [49]. The MIA model is associated with phenotypic changes in the sensory afferents; for example, mRNA expression of the α2δ-1 subunit of calcium channels is increased in ipsilateral L3 and L4 DRG at 14 days in the MIA model [45]. These changes appear to be functionally relevant as blockade of spinal voltage-gated calcium channels 2.2 ($Ca_v2.2$) attenuates mechanically evoked spinal neuronal responses in MIA-, but not saline-, injected rats at 14 days following model induction [46]. It is noteworthy that mice lacking the inhibitory cannabinoid $CB_2$ receptor exhibited contralateral decreases in hind paw withdrawal thresholds following intra-articular injection of MIA, compared with MIA-treated wild-type littermates [29], suggesting that endogenous antinociceptive systems may limit the extent of pain responses in the MIA model.

Hind paw-evoked responses of wide dynamic range neurons in the spinal cord are facilitated at both 14 [45] and 28 days [50] after intra-articular injection of MIA in the rat. By day 28 in this model, facilitated spinal neuronal responses were significantly correlated with structural changes in the joint [50], and were associated with facilitated hind paw-evoked spinal nociceptive reflexes [27]. As well as changes in neuronal activity, spinal microglia are morphologically activated in the MIA model in both time- and dose-dependent manner [48, 58]. Microgliosis is evident in the ipsilateral spinal cord from day 7 in the MIA model, peaks at 2 weeks, and is maintained until at least 4 weeks in the rat [31, 42, 48, 58]. Alongside the recruitment of additional cell types within the spinal cord, mitogen-activated protein kinases such as extracellular signal-regulated protein kinase (ERK) and p38, which are involved in the development and maintenance of centrally mediated sensitivity, are also increased. Increased p38 phosphorylation was detected in microglia in the dorsal horn of the spinal cord 1 week after MIA injection [31], supporting an early role of spinal microglia to OA pain responses. This is further substantiated by the attenuation of MIA-induced pain responses by inhibitors of microglial activation or ERK1/2 kinase [31]. Neuronal ERK1/2 phosphorylation is significantly increased in the dorsal horn at later time points (2 weeks) in the MIA model. In contrast to microglia, astrocytes are not activated in the spinal cord until 4 weeks after MIA model induction [48]. Astrocytes may, therefore, have more important roles in established OA pain, and drugs targeting astrocytes should be tested at later time points in these models. Although there have been a limited number of studies of the supraspinal alterations in models of OA pain, a 5-HT3 receptor antagonist enhanced mechanically and thermally evoked responses of spinal neurons in the model of OA pain, compared with saline controls [45]. These data support a contribution of 5-HT3-mediated descending facilitation to nociceptive responses in the MIA model [45].

## CONCLUSION

While it is widely accepted that no single animal model of OA can accurately mimic the clinical disease, these models can be used to make valuable advances in our understanding of mechanisms underlying OA pain. Chemical models of OA may have some advantages over surgical models, including being less invasive, rapid in onset, and not requiring sham-operated control. However, which models of OA most closely reflect the mechanisms of OA pain in people remains the subject of considerable debate. Given the complexity of OA and the previous difficulties in the translation of preclinical findings to the clinical setting, it is prudent to investigate the effects of specific treatments in more than one model of OA pain. For example, we have recently reported that pharmacological inhibition of the TrkA receptor produced robust antinociceptive effects in both the MIA and MNX models of OA pain [40], mirroring the robust analgesic effects of anti-NGF strategies seen in clinical trials [30]. The combination of surgical models in animals with a genetic susceptibility for OA-like pathology is likely to provide important additional advances in the future. Similarly, animal models of OA incorporating risk factors for OA, such as obesity and metabolic syndrome, may also generate more clinically relevant models of OA. Finally, a robust study design is essential to optimize translational validity. In our recent systematic review and meta-analysis of the reporting of analgesic efficacy in models of OA, we identified study design with respect to behavioral measures, limited study quality, and publication bias as factors that contribute to low specificity and reduce clinical predictive value [55].

## REFERENCES


1. Ahmed AS, Li J, Erlandsson-Harris H, Stark A, Bakalkin G, Ahmed M. Suppression of pain and joint destruction by inhibition of the proteasome system in experimental osteoarthritis. Pain 2012;153:18–26.
2. Allen KD, Griffin TM, Rodriguiz RM, Wetsel WC, Kraus VB, Huebner JL, Boyd LM, Setton LA. Decreased physical function and increased pain sensitivity in mice deficient for type IX collagen. Arthritis Rheum 2009;60:2684–93.
3. Arendt-Nielsen L, Nie H, Laursen MB, Laursen BS, Madeleine P, Simonsen OH, Graven-Nielsen T. Sensitization in patients with painful knee osteoarthritis. Pain 2010;149:573–81.
4. Ashraf S, Mapp PI, Burston J, Bennett AJ, Chapman V, Walsh DA. Augmented pain behavioural responses to intra-articular injection of nerve growth factor in two animal models of osteoarthritis. Ann Rheum Dis 2014;73:1710–18.

5. Ashraf S, Mapp PI, Walsh DA. Contributions of angiogenesis to inflammation, joint damage, and pain in a rat model of osteoarthritis. Arthritis Rheum 2011;63:2700–10.
6. Bendele AM. Animal models of osteoarthritis. J Musculoskelet Neuronal Interact 2001;1:363–76.
7. Bove SE, Flatters SJ, Inglis JJ, Mantyh PW. New advances in musculoskeletal pain. Brain Res Rev 2009;60:187–201.
8. Bullock CM, Wookey P, Bennett A, Mobasheri A, Dickerson I, Kelly S. Peripheral calcitonin gene-related peptide receptor activation and mechanical sensitization of the joint in rat models of osteoarthritis pain. Arthritis Rheumatol 2014;66:2188–200.
9. Chen M, Lichtler AC, Sheu TJ, Xie C, Zhang X, O'Keefe RJ, Chen D. Generation of a transgenic mouse model with chondrocyte-specific and tamoxifen-inducible expression of Cre recombinase. Genesis 2007;45:44–50.
10. Combe R, Bramwell S, Field MJ. The monosodium iodoacetate model of osteoarthritis: a model of chronic nociceptive pain in rats? Neurosci Lett 2004;370:236–40.
11. Daans M, Luyten FP, Lories RJ. GDF5 deficiency in mice is associated with instability-driven joint damage, gait and subchondral bone changes. Ann Rheum Dis 2011;70:208–13.
12. Dakin H, Gray A, Fitzpatrick R, Maclennan G, Murray D, Group KATT. Rationing of total knee replacement: a cost-effectiveness analysis on a large trial data set. BMJ Open 2012;2:e000332.
13. Felson DT, Niu J, Guermazi A, Roemer F, Aliabadi P, Clancy M, Torner J, Lewis CE, Nevitt MC. Correlation of the development of knee pain with enlarging bone marrow lesions on magnetic resonance imaging. Arthritis Rheum 2007;56:2986–92.
14. Ferland CE, Laverty S, Beaudry F, Vachon P. Gait analysis and pain response of two rodent models of osteoarthritis. Pharmacol Biochem Behav 2011;97:603–10.
15. Gaitan G, Herrero JF. Subanalgesic doses of dexketoprofen and HCT-2037 (nitrodexketoprofen) enhance fentanyl antinociception in monoarthritic rats. Pharmacol Biochem Behav 2005;80:327–32.
16. Gauldie SD, McQueen DS, Clarke CJ, Chessell IP. A robust model of adjuvant-induced chronic unilateral arthritis in two mouse strains. J Neurosci Methods 2004;139:281–91.
17. Glyn-Jones S, Palmer AJ, Agricola R, Price AJ, Vincent TL, Weinans H, Carr AJ. Osteoarthritis. Lancet 2015;386:376–87.
18. Guzman RE, Evans MG, Bove S, Morenko B, Kilgore K. Mono-iodoacetate-induced histologic changes in subchondral bone and articular cartilage of rat femorotibial joints: an animal model of osteoarthritis. Toxicol Pathol 2003;31:619–24.
19. Han JS, Bird GC, Li W, Jones J, Neugebauer V. Computerized analysis of audible and ultrasonic vocalizations of rats as a standardized measure of pain-related behavior. J Neurosci Methods 2005;141:261–9.
20. Hannan MT, Felson DT, Pincus T. Analysis of the discordance between radiographic changes and knee pain in osteoarthritis of the knee. J Rheumatol 2000;27:1513–7.

21. Harvey VL, Dickenson AH. Behavioural and electrophysiological characterisation of experimentally induced osteoarthritis and neuropathy in C57Bl/6 mice. Mol Pain 2009;5:18.
22. Hong Y, Ji H, Wei H. Topical ketanserin attenuates hyperalgesia and inflammation in arthritis in rats. Pain 2006;124:27–33.
23. Hsieh GC, Chandran P, Salyers AK, Pai M, Zhu CZ, Wensink EJ, Witte DG, Miller TR, Mikusa JP, Baker SJ, et al. H4 receptor antagonism exhibits antinociceptive effects in inflammatory and neuropathic pain models in rats. Pharmacol Biochem Behav 2010;95:41–50.
24. Hsieh GC, Honore P, Pai M, Wensink EJ, Chandran P, Salyers AK, Wetter JM, Zhao C, Liu H, Decker MW, et al. Antinociceptive effects of histamine H3 receptor antagonist in the preclinical models of pain in rats and the involvement of central noradrenergic systems. Brain Res 2010;1354:74–84.
25. Inglis JJ, McNamee KE, Chia SL, Essex D, Feldmann M, Williams RO, Hunt SP, Vincent T. Regulation of pain sensitivity in experimental osteoarthritis by the endogenous peripheral opioid system. Arthritis Rheum 2008;58:3110–19.
26. Karsdal MA, Bay-Jensen AC, Lories RJ, Abramson S, Spector T, Pastoureau P, Christiansen C, Attur M, Henriksen K, Goldring SR, Kraus V. The coupling of bone and cartilage turnover in osteoarthritis: opportunities for bone antiresorptives and anabolics as potential treatments? Ann Rheum Dis 2014;73: 336–48.
27. Kelly S, Dobson KL, Harris J. Spinal nociceptive reflexes are sensitized in the monosodium iodoacetate model of osteoarthritis pain in the rat. Osteoarthritis Cartilage/OARS, Osteoarthritis Res Soc 2013;21:1327–35.
28. Kelly S, Dunham JP, Murray F, Read S, Donaldson LF, Lawson SN. Spontaneous firing in C-fibers and increased mechanical sensitivity in A-fibers of knee joint-associated mechanoreceptive primary afferent neurones during MIA-induced osteoarthritis in the rat. Osteoarthritis Cartilage/OARS, Osteoarthritis Res Soc 2012;20:305–13.
29. La Porta C, Bura SA, Aracil-Fernandez A, Manzanares J, Maldonado R. Role of CB1 and CB2 cannabinoid receptors in the development of joint pain induced by monosodium iodoacetate. Pain 2013;154:160–74.
30. Lane NE, Schnitzer TJ, Birbara CA, Mokhtarani M, Shelton DL, Smith MD, Brown MT. Tanezumab for the treatment of pain from osteoarthritis of the knee. N Engl J Med 2010;363:1521–31.
31. Lee Y, Pai M, Brederson JD, Wilcox D, Hsieh G, Jarvis MF, Bitner RS. Monosodium iodoacetate-induced joint pain is associated with increased phosphorylation of mitogen activated protein kinases in the rat spinal cord. Mol Pain 2011;7:39.
32. Malfait AM, Ritchie J, Gil AS, Austin JS, Hartke J, Qin W, Tortorella MD, Mogil JS. ADAMTS-5 deficient mice do not develop mechanical allodynia associated with osteoarthritis following medial meniscal destabilization. Osteoarthritis Cartilage/OARS, Osteoarthritis Res Soc 2010;18:572–80.
33. Mapp PI, Sagar DR, Ashraf S, Burston JJ, Suri S, Chapman V, Walsh DA. Differences in structural and pain phenotypes in the sodium monoiodoacetate and

meniscal transection models of osteoarthritis. Osteoarthritis Cartilage/OARS, Osteoarthritis Res Soc 2013;21(9):1336–45.

34. McDougall JJ, Andruski B, Schuelert N, Hallgrímsson B, Matyas JR. Unravelling the relationship between age, nociception and joint destruction in naturally occurring osteoarthritis of Dunkin Hartley guinea pigs. Pain 2009;141:222–32.
35. McDougall JJ, Barin AK, McDougall CM. Loss of vasomotor responsiveness to the mu-opioid receptor ligand endomorphin-1 in adjuvant monoarthritic rat knee joints. Am J Physiol Regul Integr Comp Physiol 2004;286:R634–41.
36. Min SS, Han JS, Kim YI, Na HS, Yoon YW, Hong SK, Han HC. A novel method for convenient assessment of arthritic pain in voluntarily walking rats. Neurosci Lett 2001;308:95–8.
37. Murray CJ, Vos T, Lozano R, Naghavi M, Flaxman AD, Michaud C, Ezzati M, Shibuya K, Salomon JA, Abdalla S, et al. Disability-adjusted life years (DALYs) for 291 diseases and injuries in 21 regions, 1990–2010: a systematic analysis for the Global Burden of Disease Study 2010. Lancet 2012;380:2197–223.
38. National Clinical Guideline Centre, National Institute for Health and Clinical Excellence: Guidance. Osteoarthritis:Osteoarthritis: and Management in Adults. London: National Institute for Health and Care Excellence (UK); 2014
39. Neugebauer V, Schaible HG. Evidence for a central component in the sensitization of spinal neurons with joint input during development of acute arthritis in cat's knee. J Neurophysiol 1990;64:299–311.
40. Nwosu LN, Mapp PI, Chapman V, Walsh DA. Blocking the tropomyosin receptor kinase A (TrkA) receptor inhibits pain behaviour in two rat models of osteoarthritis. Ann Rheum Dis 2015. doi:10.1136/annrheumdis-2014-207203.
41. Ogbonna AC, Clark AK, Gentry C, Hobbs C, Malcangio M. Pain-like behaviour and spinal changes in the monosodium iodoacetate model of osteoarthritis in C57Bl/6 mice. Eur J Pain 2013;17:514–26.
42. Orita S, Ishikawa T, Miyagi M, Ochiai N, Inoue G, Eguchi Y, Kamoda H, Arai G, Suzuki M, Sakuma Y, Oikawa Y. Percutaneously absorbed NSAIDs attenuate local production of proinflammatory cytokines and suppress the expression of c-Fos in the spinal cord of a rodent model of knee osteoarthritis. J Orthop Sci 2012;17:77–86.
43. Pavlaković G, Petzke F. The role of quantitative sensory testing in the evaluation of musculoskeletal pain conditions. Curr Rheumatol Rep 2010;12:455–61.
44. Poole R, Blake S, Buschmann M, Goldring S, Laverty S, Lockwood S, Matyas J, McDougall J, Pritzker K, Rudolphi K, van den Berg W. Recommendations for the use of preclinical models in the study and treatment of osteoarthritis. Osteoarthritis Cartilage/OARS, Osteoarthritis Res Soc 2010;18:S10–6.
45. Rahman W, Bauer CS, Bannister K, Vonsy JL, Dolphin AC, Dickenson AH. Descending serotonergic facilitation and the antinociceptive effects of pregabalin in a rat model of osteoarthritic pain. Mol Pain 2009;5:45.
46. Rahman W, Patel R, Dickenson AH. Electrophysiological evidence for voltage-gated calcium channel 2 (Cav2) modulation of mechano- and thermosensitive spinal neuronal responses in a rat model of osteoarthritis. Neuroscience 2015;305:76–85.

47. Rountree RB, Schoor M, Chen H, Marks ME, Harley V, Mishina Y, Kingsley DM. BMP receptor signaling is required for postnatal maintenance of articular cartilage. PLoS Biol 2004;2:e355.
48. Sagar DR, Burston JJ, Hathway GJ, Woodhams SG, Pearson RG, Bennett AJ, Kendall DA, Scammell BE, Chapman V. The contribution of spinal glial cells to chronic pain behaviour in the monosodium iodoacetate model of osteoarthritic pain. Mol Pain 2011;7:88.
49. Sagar DR, Nwosu L, Walsh DA, Chapman V. Dissecting the contribution of knee joint NGF to spinal nociceptive sensitization in a model of OA pain in the rat. Osteoarthritis Cartilage/OARS, Osteoarthritis Res Soc 2015;23:906–13.
50. Sagar DR, Staniaszek LE, Okine BN, Woodhams S, Norris LM, Pearson RG, Garle MJ, Alexander SP, Bennett AJ, Barrett DA, Kendall DA. Tonic modulation of spinal hyperexcitability by the endocannabinoid receptor system in a rat model of osteoarthritis pain. Arthritis Rheum 2010;62:3666–76.
51. Seino D, Tokunaga A, Tachibana T, Yoshiya S, Dai Y, Obata K, Yamanaka H, Kobayashi K, Noguchi K. The role of ERK signaling and the P2X receptor on mechanical pain evoked by movement of inflamed knee joint. Pain 2006;123:193–203.
52. Sluka KA, Skyba DA, Radhakrishnan R, Leeper BJ, Wright A. Joint mobilization reduces hyperalgesia associated with chronic muscle and joint inflammation in rats. J Pain 2006;7:602–7.
53. Sluka KA, Westlund KN. Behavioral and immunohistochemical changes in an experimental arthritis model in rats. Pain 1993;55:367–77.
54. Staton PC, Wilson AW, Bountra C, Chessell IP, Day NC. Changes in dorsal root ganglion CGRP expression in a chronic inflammatory model of the rat knee joint: differential modulation by rofecoxib and paracetamol. Eur J Pain 2007;11:283–9.
55. Suokas AK, Sagar DR, Mapp PI, Chapman V, Walsh DA. Design, study quality and evidence of analgesic efficacy in studies of drugs in models of OA pain: a systematic review and a meta-analysis. Osteoarthritis Cartilage/OARS, Osteoarthritis Res Soc 2014;22:1207–23.
56. Suokas AK, Walsh DA, McWilliams DF, Condon L, Moreton B, Wylde V, Arendt-Nielsen L, Zhang W. Quantitative sensory testing in painful osteoarthritis: a systematic review and meta-analysis. Osteoarthritis Cartilage/OARS, Osteoarthritis Res Soc 2012;20:1075–85.
57. Teeple E, Jay GD, Elsaid KA, Fleming BC. Animal models of osteoarthritis: challenges of model selection and analysis. AAPS J 2013;15(2):438–46.
58. Thakur M, Rahman W, Hobbs C, Dickenson AH, Bennett DL. Characterisation of a peripheral neuropathic component of the rat monoiodoacetate model of osteoarthritis. PLoS One 2012;7:e33730.
59. Tonussi CR, Ferreira SH. Rat knee-joint carrageenan incapacitation test: an objective screen for central and peripheral analgesics. Pain 1992;48:421–7.
60. Upadhyay J, Baker SJ, Rajagovindan R, Hart M, Chandran P, Hooker BA, Cassar S, Mikusa JP, Tovcimak A, Wald MJ, Joshi SK. Pharmacological modulation of brain activity in a preclinical model of osteoarthritis. Neuroimage 2013;64:341–55.
61. Valdes AM, Spector TD. The clinical relevance of genetic susceptibility to osteoarthritis. Best Pract Res Clin Rheumatol 2010;24(1):3–14.

62. Vincent TL, Williams RO, Maciewicz R, Silman A, Garside P, Arthritis Research UK Animal Models Working Group. Mapping pathogenesis of arthritis through small animal models. Rheumatology (Oxford) 2012;51(11):1931–41.
63. Vos T, Flaxman AD, Naghavi M, Lozano R, Michaud C, Ezzati M, Shibuya K, Salomon JA, Abdalla S, Aboyans V, et al. Years lived with disability (YLDs) for 1160 sequelae of 289 diseases and injuries 1990–2010: a systematic analysis for the Global Burden of Disease Study 2010. Lancet 2012;380(9859):2163–96.
64. Wu Q, Henry JL. Changes in Abeta non-nociceptive primary sensory neurons in a rat model of osteoarthritis pain. Mol Pain 2010;6:37.
65. Wu Q, Henry JL. Peripheral drive in Aα/β-fiber neurons is altered in a rat model of osteoarthritis: changes in following frequency and recovery from inactivation. J Pain Res 2013;6:207–21.
66. Yu YC, Koo ST, Kim CH, Lyu Y, Grady JJ, Chung JM. Two variables that can be used as pain indices in experimental animal models of arthritis. J Neurosci Methods 2002;115(1):107–13.
67. Zhang L, Hoff AO, Wimalawansa SJ, Cote GJ, Gagel RF, Westlund KN. Arthritic calcitonin/alpha calcitonin gene-related peptide knockout mice have reduced nociceptive hypersensitivity. Pain 2001;89:265–73.
68. Zhang W, Doherty M, Peat G, Bierma-Zeinstra MA, Arden NK, Bresnihan B, Herrero-Beaumont G, Kirschner S, Leeb BF, Lohmander LS, et al. EULAR evidence-based recommendations for the diagnosis of knee osteoarthritis. Ann Rheum Dis 2010;69(3):483–9.

CHAPTER 4

# Joint Pain in Pet Dogs and Cats

*B. Duncan X. Lascelles, Margaret E. Gruen, and John F. Innes*

Arthritidies are common in companion animals, and joint pain, particularly associated with osteoarthritis (OA), is common in companion animals such as dogs, cats, and horses. It results in impairment in mobility and performance of activities and is associated with spontaneous and induced pain. Arthritis in dogs [21] and cats [28] has been reviewed in detail, including current knowledge about etiology, pathogenesis, diagnosis, and treatment.

In pet dogs, OA is a common condition possibly affecting a quarter of the population [21]. In pet cats, radiographic evidence of OA/degenerative joint disease (DJD) is apparent in up to 90% of all cats [32], with an estimated 50% of these having clinical signs of impairment due to joint pain, such as changes in mobility, particularly gait, jumping, and use of stairs [24]. Other painful DJDs such as the immune-mediated arthropathies occur in dogs and cats, but less frequently than the inflammatory arthropathies (such as rheumatoid arthritis) in humans.

## ETIOLOGY AND PATHOPHYSIOLOGY

In contrast to humans, OA in dogs is mainly due to developmental orthopedic diseases—hip dysplasia, elbow dysplasia, osteochondrosis dissecans, nontraumatic cranial cruciate ligament degeneration—and so is considered an early onset disease and a lifelong disease. The joints most commonly affected are the hip, stifle, and elbow [21].

Less is known about the etiology of OA in cats than in dogs, but the degenerative disease process appears very similar to that of other species [10, 13]. The joints most commonly affected are the hip, stifle, tarsus, and elbow. For feline synovial joints, there are several recognized and postulated primary and secondary causes of joint degeneration. DJDs associated with Scottish Fold osteochondrodysplasia [36], mucopolysaccharidosis [27], and age-related cartilage degeneration have all been described as primary DJD. Postulated secondary causes of DJD in cats are congenital, trauma, infectious and inflammatory, nutritional, and immune-mediated [28], although there is little evidence for many of these causes. Indeed, one of the most common causes of elbow OA in the dog is fragmented coronoid process (part of the developmental elbow dysplasia), but recent evidence indicates that this does not occur in the cat [13]. Conversely, hip dysplasia occurs in cats, as it does in dogs, and is associated with OA [23].

In both cats and dogs, all tissues of the joint are involved in the degenerative process, and pain is commonly associated with the disease, although, as in humans, pain cannot be predicted by radiographic appearance [29]. Radiography does, however, predict alterations in range of motion [29]. Peripheral and central nervous system plasticity associated with joint pain has been demonstrated in both cats [17] and dogs [47] and is thought to contribute to the overall pain state.

Pain associated with joint disease results in impaired or altered mobility, impaired ability to perform activities, and altered behavior. In dogs, it has been shown to disrupt sleep [25] and is thought to impair cognitive function. In both species, the multidimensional effects of pain appear similar to the effects in humans [24, 45].

## CLINICAL SIGNS AND DIAGNOSIS

In clinical veterinary practice, diagnosis is centered on four elements:

1. Owner-reported activity impairment. Although more readily detected in dogs, several clinical metrology instruments for use in the clinical setting (as well as for clinical research) have been

developed to measure this in dogs (Canine Brief Pain Inventory [CBPI] [5]; Liverpool Osteoarthritis in Dogs [LOAD] [45]) and also in cats (Feline Musculoskeletal Pain Index [FMPI] [1, 15]).

2. Pain on manipulation of affected joints during an orthopedic evaluation, with pain being measured as a behavioral response of varying intensity.
3. Radiographic evidence of OA (effusion; osteophytes; subchondral sclerosis; joint-associated mineralization).
4. Gait and movement evaluation, or performance testing, such as observing gait at walk and trot (dogs), fluidity of movement in the room, and ability to jump onto a chair or down from the examination table (cats).

Additionally, synovial fluid analysis is sometimes performed. This is infrequently performed unless the clinical picture and examination findings suggest an inflammatory arthropathy such as an immune-medicated arthritis.

In referral centers or in the comparative research setting, the effects of pain can be measured in both species by:

- Measuring limb use (kinetic variables measured using force plates or pressure sensitive walkways) [30]
- Measuring spontaneous activity through accelerometry [8]
- Measuring central plasticity through quantitative sensory threshold testing [9, 47]

## TREATMENT

Because of a relative paucity of evidence-based information regarding treatment of dogs and cats, much of the current clinical approach to treatment is based on information borrowed from human medicine. The dominant approach to treatment of joint pain associated with OA in both dogs [21] and cats [28] revolves around medical management, with surgery, though available, being used infrequently. The same is true for the inflammatory arthropathies, although there is emphasis by clinicians on detecting and removing the underlying cause if identifiable. Most joint pain is treated in primary practice settings, as opposed to being treated in referral centers by board-specialized veterinarians. Increasingly, confounding comorbidities are a focus of the treatment of OA, such as obesity management. Just as with humans, dogs and cats are increasingly becoming obese, and weight management is a crucial part of the management of OA.

## Dogs

- A multimodal drug and nondrug approach is recommended to manage OA-associated pain [40].
- The only class of drug approved by the U.S. Food and Drug Administration (FDA) Center for Veterinary Medicine is the nonsteroidal anti-inflammatory drug (NSAID) class (several approved), though other classes (caninized anti-nerve growth factor [14, 33] and prostaglandin E4 receptor antagonists [piprants], among others) are in development.
- Local (intra-articular) therapies are occasionally used, and several drugs (such as capsaicin analogs) are in development.
- Most evidence exists for efficacy of NSAIDs, dietary modulation through omega-3 fatty acid supplementation [43], weight management, and exercise.
- Adjunctive drug therapy (amantadine, tramadol, gabapentin) is commonly employed (evidence for efficacy of amantadine [31]; limited evidence for oral tramadol, which is metabolized very differently in the dog; no evidence for gabapentin). Adjunctive nondrug therapy is also popular, such as acupuncture. Overall, there is a lack of studies evaluating these therapies.
- Physical rehabilitation (exercise, therapeutic exercise, and other physical modalities such as therapeutic laser, therapeutic ultrasound, hydrotherapy, and massage) is commonly employed.
- Surgical joint replacement is available and used in the dog (hip, stifle, and elbow).

- Combination steroid and immunosuppressive therapies are used in the management of immune-mediated joint pain.
- Dietary supplements are commonly used, although there is currently no evidence (other than omega-3 fatty acids) for any benefit in reducing pain.

### Cats

- A multimodal drug and nondrug approach is recommended to manage OA and DJD-associated pain [2].
- There are no FDA-approved drug treatments and only one approved drug in the European Union (an NSAID), though other classes (felinized anti-nerve growth factor and prostaglandin E4 receptor antagonists [piprant], among others) are in development.
- Most evidence exists for efficacy of NSAIDs and dietary modulation through omega-3 fatty acid supplementation [43].
- Adjunctive drug therapy (mainly gabapentin and polysulphated glycosaminoglycans) is employed, but studies evaluating these therapies are lacking.
- Surgical joint replacement is available for the hip, and other custom joint replacements have been performed.
- Non-fatty acid dietary supplements are commonly used, although there is currently no evidence for any benefit in reducing pain.

## PREVENTION

The prevention of joint disease in cats and dogs is receiving increasing attention, with both lifestyle management techniques and surgical techniques being investigated. The most dramatic evidence for a preventative measure comes from studies showing that lifetime calorie restriction (prevention of obesity) dramatically decreases the incidence of radiographic evidence of OA [22].

## USE OF COMPANION ANIMALS WITH JOINT PAIN IN TRANSLATIONAL RESEARCH

The current practice of translational biomedical research is not producing new therapeutics for use in humans, with as much as 90% of drugs entering Phase 1 studies failing to reach clinical use [11, 19]. With respect to pain, numerous reviews [3, 37, 39, 44] have highlighted a crippling lack of translation of basic research into new approved therapeutics for treatment of persistent pain in humans, and a recent review highlighted the paucity of animal models of OA [34]. Although many aspects of the translational drug development pathway have been highlighted as needing improvement, the use of highly inbred and genetically modified laboratory animals kept in homogeneous and closely regulated environments is a markedly different situation to humans, who exhibit genetic variability, have diverse diets and personal habits, and live in varied environments. The use of spontaneous painful disease in companion animals was highlighted as one of the changes that could be made to help improve translation of basic science to new therapeutics [38], and other recent reviews have highlighted the potential of spontaneous disease in companion animals in the translational paradigm, acting as a bridge between preclinical and clinical studies, with the goal of reducing the failure rates of human clinical trials, thus accelerating the approval of new therapeutics [26].

The pathophysiology of canine OA of the hip is considered to be very similar to human OA in terms of molecular changes [10], and the radiographic features are very similar (Fig. 4-1). Human knee OA is common, and the canine stifle joint is considered to be among the most similar to the human knee joint [12]. As well as the disease-process fidelity, such spontaneous models have the added benefit that these companion animals share the same environment as humans, potentially making the model more relevant than some rodent models [38]. Naturally occurring disease such as OA in dogs and cats may better reflect the complex genetic, environmental, and physiological variation present in the human population.

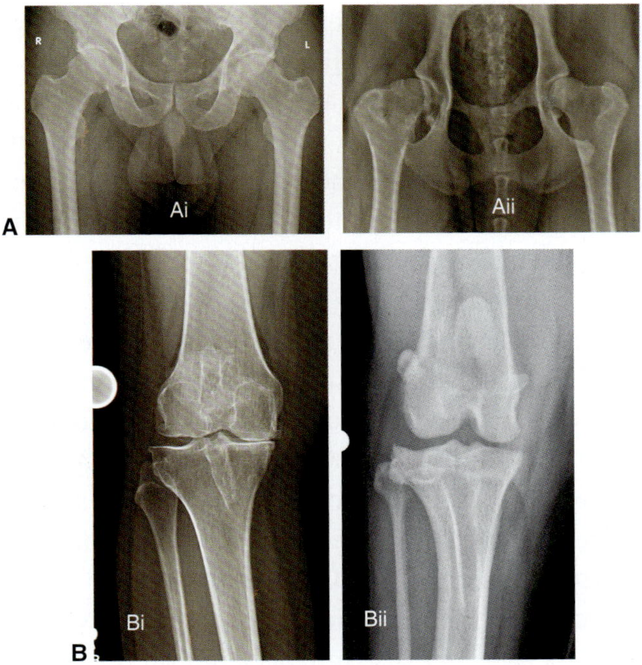


**FIGURE 4-1** **A:** Osteoarthritis (OA) in humans is very similar to the *naturally occurring disease* of OA in pet dogs and pet cats. Radiograph **Ai** depicts bilateral coxofemoral joint OA in a human subject with femoral–acetabular interference and secondary OA; radiograph **Aii** depicts bilateral coxofemoral joint OA in a dog, secondary to naturally occurring hip dysplasia in a pet dog. Both show almost identical radiographic features, with distorted femoral heads, subchondral sclerosis, and osteophytosis. **B:** Radiographs show knee OA in a human subject (**Bi**) and stifle (knee) OA in a pet dog (**Bii**), secondary to naturally occurring cranial cruciate ligament damage. Both radiographs show similar radiographic features. Additionally, the gross and histological appearance of the disease in both species is almost identical.

However, for spontaneous disease models to be used in translational research, outcome measures of the many dimensions of pain, reflecting the complexity of the disease in humans, need to be well developed. Overall, outcome measures are relatively well developed in the dog but less so in the cat. The effects of joint pain can be measured in both species by measuring changes in limb use (kinetic variables measured using force plates [41]) or pressure sensitive walkways [30]. Indeed, arthritis-induced gait changes in higher order mammals (e.g., dogs and cats) are more pronounced than in rodents, making these animals better suited for kinematic studies [35].

The effects of pain on spontaneous activity can also be measured through accelerometry [8, 18], and this may be particularly a good outcome measure in pet cats where activity is not influenced by being taken on walks [15]. Accelerometry in client-owned animals, in their home environments, has been used to show efficacy for several analgesics used in OA management.

Owner-administered clinical metrology instruments have been developed, and validated as measures of pain and impairment in performing daily activities. The most developed for dogs are the LOAD [20, 45] and the CBPI [5]. The LOAD [20, 45] is a 13-item instrument, with all items reported on a five-point Likert-type scale. Each item is scored between 0 and 4, and the item scores are summed to give an overall instrument score. The LOAD appears to cover three domains: activity/exercise, stiffness/lameness, and effect of weather [45]. The CBPI [5–7] is a two-part instrument based on the human Brief Pain Inventory; the pain severity score (CBPI PSS) is the arithmetic mean of four items scored on an 11-point (0–10) numerical scale, and the pain interference score (CBPI PIS) is the mean of six items scored similarly. Although it has been reported to measure two dimensions (pain and interference) [6], recent work suggests that it covers only one domain [45]. Subjective rating scales for quality of life have been developed for use in dogs. The Glasgow University Veterinary School questionnaire (GUVQuest) (http://theses.gla.ac.uk/3193/1/2005WisemanOrrPhd.pdf) consists of 109 descriptors rated on a scale of 1–7 and assesses pain through its impact on health-related quality of life, but use of the scale has not been published. Pain is more difficult to measure in cats, but recent work has developed the first clinical metrology instruments [1, 15].

Additionally, measures of sleep disturbance have been developed in dogs with OA [25], and measures of central plasticity through quantitative sensory threshold testing [9, 47]. Early work evaluated the repeatability of quantitative sensory threshold measures [4, 47], and two small studies have suggested the presence of central plasticity in association with cruciate ligament rupture [9] and hind limb OA [47].

Additionally, one study concluded that unilateral total hip replacement in client-owned dogs with bilateral hip OA resulted in decreased central sensitization, as measured using von Frey thresholds, 12 months after surgery [42]; however, controls were not evaluated.

Although studies have not been performed, joint pain in cats and dogs is considered to impact cognitive function, anxiety, and fear, all areas that need to be investigated in the future.

Studies in companion animals are feasible, and randomized, blinded clinical trials with sample sizes approaching those of some human clinical trials are possible [46]. Owners of companion animals are dedicated to their pets' health and willing to engage in clinical studies. Indeed, recent evidence suggests that many owners are altruistic in this respect, participating in clinical studies if the results would benefit other animals [16].

Cross-disciplinary collaboration among physicians, scientists, and veterinary clinical scientists, combined with a global multi-institutional companion animal pain research network, could facilitate the rapid and ethical in vivo evaluation of putative analgesics in these spontaneous disease models (Fig. 4-2).

One final consideration is that drug development programs will fail if their biological basis (i.e., the starting evidence) is not sound. This refers to the target. The evaluation of tissue from naturally occurring disease states may provide vital information in the translational jigsaw—information about the *neurobiology of pain in the natural disease state*. This tissue is available; peripheral tissue can be readily obtained from the millions of joint surgeries performed each year on pet dogs, and central nervous system tissues are available from the thousands of dogs with OA-associated pain that are euthanized each year. Indeed, the presence of OA-associated pain and mobility impairment is one of the most common reasons for euthanasia in pet dogs. So far, the assumption has been that the mechanisms discovered in a rodent model are relevant to the natural disease state. An informative approach would be to ask "what mechanisms are altered in the natural disease state?" Additionally, as phenotyping of these spontaneous models develops further, this, combined with the inherent smaller degree of genetic variability in dogs compared with humans, could lead to the discovery

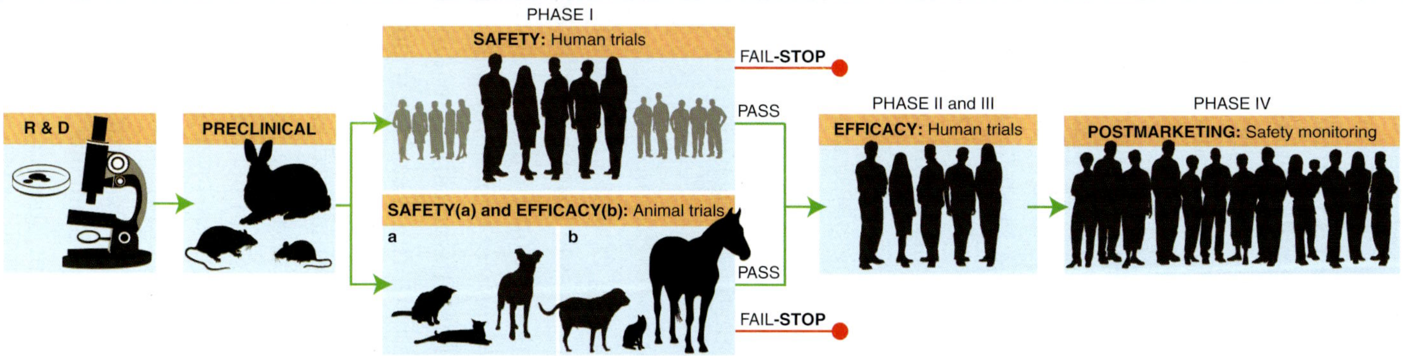


**FIGURE 4-2** In classic therapeutic development, drug candidates are discovered in the Research and Development (R&D) phase, and candidates are further narrowed down and chosen during preclinical investigations in rodent testing and rodent models of pain. The most promising candidate(s) is moved forward into Phase 1 human studies to primarily assess safety, and then into Phase 2 and 3 efficacy (and further safety) studies. Most drugs fail in the transition from safety-focused studies to efficacy-focused studies. One obvious place that naturally occurring joint pain in pets could help in the translational process is to assist in the "go/no-go" decision-making process early on by testing efficacy in a relevant model—that is, a naturally occurring disease state that is the same as the target disease in humans. These studies would be performed in owned pet animals, and these studies could be done in parallel with Phase 1 human studies, thus limiting the extension of drug development timelines, if any. An approach such as this could help to prevent nonefficacious drugs going into expensive human clinical studies. If a therapeutic candidate failed either Phase 1 studies or efficacy studies in pets with naturally occurring disease, the development would be stopped. A putative therapeutic that both passed human Phase 1 studies and showed efficacy in naturally occurring conditions in companion animals would move to Phase 2/3 studies.

of genetic and epigenetic characteristics that protect against pain or promote pain.

## ACKNOWLEDGMENTS

The authors thank Dr. Jimi Cook and Dr. Simon Roe for the radiographs used in Fig. 4-1, and Alice Harvey of NC State College of Veterinary Medicine's Media and Design unit.

### REFERENCES

1. Benito J, Hansen B, DePuy V, Davidson GS, Thomson A, Simpson W, Roe S, Hardie E, Lascelles BDX. Feline musculoskeletal pain index: responsiveness and testing of criterion validity. J Vet Intern Med 2013;27:474–82.
2. Bennett D, Zainal Ariffin SMB, Johnston P. Osteoarthritis in the cat: 2. How should it be managed and treated? J Feline Med Surg 2012;14:76–84.
3. Borsook D, Hargreaves R, Bountra C, Porreca F. Lost but making progress: where will new analgesic drugs come from? Sci Transl Med 2014;6:249sr3.
4. Briley JD, Williams MD, Freire M, Griffith EH, Lascelles BDX. Feasibility and repeatability of cold and mechanical quantitative sensory testing in normal dogs. Vet J 2014;199:245–50.
5. Brown DC, Boston RC, Coyne JC. Ability of the canine brief pain inventory to detect response to treatment in dogs with osteoarthritis. J Am Vet Med Assoc 2008;233(8):1278–83.
6. Brown DC, Boston RC, Coyne JC, Farrar JT. Development and psychometric testing of an instrument designed to measure chronic pain in dogs with osteoarthritis. Am J Vet Res 2007;68:631–37.
7. Brown DC, Boston RC, Farrar JT. Comparison of force plate gait analysis and owner assessment of pain using the canine brief pain inventory in dogs with osteoarthritis. J Vet Intern Med 2013;27:22–30.
8. Brown DC, Boston RC, Farrar JT. Use of an activity monitor to detect response to treatment in dogs with osteoarthritis. J Am Vet Med Assoc 2010;237:66–70.
9. Brydges NM, Argyle DJ, Mosley JR, Duncan JC, Fleetwood-Walker S, Clements DN. Clinical assessments of increased sensory sensitivity in dogs with cranial cruciate ligament rupture. Vet J 2012;193:545–50.
10. Clements DN, Carter SD, Innes JF, Ollier WER, Day PJR. Analysis of normal and osteoarthritic canine cartilage mRNA expression by quantitative polymerase chain reaction. Arthritis Res Ther 2006;8:R158.
11. Contopoulos-Ioannidis DG, Ntzani E, Ioannidis JPA. Translation of highly promising basic science research into clinical applications. Am J Med 2003;114:477–84.

12. Cook JL, Kuroki K, Visco D, Pelletier JP, Schulz L, Lafeber FPJG. The OARSI histopathology initiative: recommendations for histological assessments of osteoarthritis in the dog. Osteoarthritis Cartilage 2010;18:S66–79.
13. Freire M, Meuten D, Lascelles D. Pathology of articular cartilage and synovial membrane from elbow joints with and without degenerative joint disease in domestic cats. Vet Pathol 2014;51:968–78.
14. Gearing DP, Virtue ER, Gearing RP, Drew AC. A fully caninised anti-NGF monoclonal antibody for pain relief in dogs. BMC Vet Res 2013;9:226.
15. Gruen ME, Griffith EH, Thomson AE, Simpson W, Lascelles BDX. Criterion validation testing of clinical metrology instruments for measuring degenerative joint disease associated mobility impairment in cats. PLoS One 2015;10:e0131839.
16. Gruen ME, Jiamachello KN, Thomson A, Lascelles BDX. Clinical trials involving cats: what factors affect owner participation? J Feline Med Surg 2014;16: 727–35.
17. Guillot M, Taylor PM, Rialland P, Klinck MP, Martel-Pelletier J, Pelletier J-P, Troncy E. Evoked temporal summation in cats to highlight central sensitization related to osteoarthritis-associated chronic pain: a preliminary study. PLoS One 2014;9:e97347.
18. Hansen BD, Lascelles BDX, Keene BW, Adams AK, Thomson AE. Evaluation of an accelerometer for at-home monitoring of spontaneous activity in dogs. Am J Vet Res 2007;68:468–75.
19. Hay M, Thomas DW, Craighead JL, Economides C, Rosenthal J. Clinical development success rates for investigational drugs. Nat Biotechnol 2014;32:40–51.
20. Hercock CA, Pinchbeck G, Giejda A, Clegg PD, Innes JF. Validation of a client-based clinical metrology instrument for the evaluation of canine elbow osteoarthritis. J Small Anim Pract 2009;50:266–271.
21. Innes JF. Arthritis. In: Tobias KM, Johnston ST, editors. Veterinary surgery: small animal, Vol. 1. St. Louis: Elsevier Saunders; 2012. p. 1078–111.
22. Kealy RD, Lawler DF, Ballam JM, Mantz SL, Biery DN, Greeley EH, Lust G, Segre M, Smith GK, Stowe HD. Effects of diet restriction on life span and age-related changes in dogs. J Am Vet Med Assoc 2002;220:1315–20.
23. Keller GG, Reed AL, Lattimer JC, Corley EA. Hip dysplasia: a feline population study. Vet Radiol Ultrasound 1999;40:460–64.
24. Klinck MP, Frank D, Guillot M, Troncy E. Owner-perceived signs and veterinary diagnosis in 50 cases of feline osteoarthritis. Can Vet J 2012;53:1181–86.
25. Knazovicky D, Tomas A, Motsinger-Reif A, Lascelles BDX. Initial evaluation of nighttime restlessness in a naturally occurring canine model of osteoarthritis pain. Peer J 2015;3:e772.
26. Kol A, Arzi B, Athanasiou KA, Farmer DL, Nolta JA, Rebhun RB, Chen X, Griffiths LG, Verstraete FJM, Murphy CJ, Borjesson DL. Companion animals: translational scientist's new best friends. Sci Transl Med 2015;7:308ps21.
27. Konde LJ, Thrall MA, Gasper P, Dial SM, McBiles K, Colgan S, Haskins M. Radiographically visualized skeletal changes associated with mucopolysaccharidosis VI in cats. Vet Radiol 1987;28:223–8.
28. Lascelles BDX. Feline degenerative joint disease. Vet Surg 2010;39:2–13.

29. Lascelles BDX, Dong Y-H, Marcellin-Little DJ, Thomson A, Wheeler S, Correa M. Relationship of orthopedic examination, goniometric measurements, and radiographic signs of degenerative joint disease in cats. BMC Vet Res 2012;8:10.
30. Lascelles BDX, Freire M, Roe SC, DePuy V, Smith E, Marcellin-Little DJ. Evaluation of functional outcome after BFX total hip replacement using a pressure sensitive walkway. Vet Surg 2010;39:71–77.
31. Lascelles BDX, Gaynor JS, Smith ES, Roe SC, Marcellin-Little DJ, Davidson G, Boland E, Carr J. Amantadine in a multimodal analgesic regimen for alleviation of refractory osteoarthritis pain in dogs. J Vet Intern Med 2008;22:53–9.
32. Lascelles BDX, Henry JB III, Brown J, Robertson I, Sumrell AT, Simpson W, Wheeler S, Hansen BD, Zamprogno H, Freire M, Pease A. Cross-sectional study of the prevalence of radiographic degenerative joint disease in domesticated cats. Vet Surg 2010;39:535–44.
33. Lascelles BDX, Knazovicky D, Case B, Freire M, Innes JF, Drew AC, Gearing DP. A canine-specific anti-nerve growth factor antibody alleviates pain and improves mobility and function in dogs with degenerative joint disease-associated pain. BMC Vet Res 2015;11:101.
34. Malfait A-M, Little CB. On the predictive utility of animal models of osteoarthritis. Arthritis Res Ther 2015;17:225.
35. Malfait AM, Little CB, McDougall JJ. A commentary on modelling osteoarthritis pain in small animals. Osteoarthritis Cartilage 2013;21:1316–26.
36. Malik R, Allan GS, Howlett CR, Thompson DE, James G, McWhirter C, Kendall K. Osteochondrodysplasia in Scottish Fold cats. Aust Vet J 1999;77:85–92.
37. Mogil JS. Animal models of pain: progress and challenges. Nat Rev Neurosci 2009;10:283–94.
38. Percie du Sert N, Rice ASC. Improving the translation of analgesic drugs to the clinic: animal models of neuropathic pain. Br J Pharmacol 2014;171:2951–63.
39. Rice ASC, Cimino-Brown D, Eisenach JC, Kontinen VK, Lacroix-Fralish ML, Machin I, Preclinical Pain Consortium, Mogil JS, Stöhr T. Animal models and the prediction of efficacy in clinical trials of analgesic drugs: a critical appraisal and call for uniform reporting standards. Pain 2008;139:243–47.
40. Rychel JK. Diagnosis and treatment of osteoarthritis. Top Companion Anim Med 2010;25:20–5.
41. Stejskal M, Torres BT, Sandberg GS, Sapora JA, Dover RK, Budsberg SC. Variability of vertical ground reaction forces collected with one and two force plates in healthy dogs. Vet Comp Orthop Traumatol 2015;28:318–22.
42. Tomas A, Marcellin-Little DJ, Roe SC, Motsinger-Reif A, Lascelles BDX. Relationship between mechanical thresholds and limb use in dogs with coxofemoral joint OA-associated pain and the modulating effects of pain alleviation from total hip replacement on mechanical thresholds. Vet Surg 2014;43:542–48.
43. Vandeweerd JM, Coisnon C, Clegg P, Cambier C, Pierson A, Hontoir F, Saegerman C, Gustin P, Buczinski S. Systematic review of efficacy of nutraceuticals to alleviate clinical signs of osteoarthritis. J Vet Intern Med 2012;26:448–56.
44. Vierck CJ, Hansson PT, Yezierski RP. Clinical and pre-clinical pain assessment: are we measuring the same thing? Pain 2008;135:7–10.

45. Walton MB, Cowderoy E, Lascelles D, Innes JF. Evaluation of construct and criterion validity for the "Liverpool Osteoarthritis in Dogs" (LOAD) clinical metrology instrument and comparison to two other instruments. PLoS One 2013;8:e58125.
46. Walton MB, Cowderoy EC, Wustefeld-Janssens B, Lascelles BDX, Innes JF. Mavacoxib and meloxicam for canine osteoarthritis: a randomised clinical comparator trial. Vet Rec 2014;175:280.
47. Williams MD, Kirkpatrick AE, Griffith E, Benito J, Hash J, Lascelles BDX. Feasibility and repeatability of thermal quantitative sensory testing in normal dogs and dogs with hind limb osteoarthritis-associated pain. Vet J 2014;199:63–7.

CHAPTER 5

# Joint Biochemistry for Cartilage, Bone, Cartilage Degradation, Bone Remodeling, and Inflammation in Osteoarthritis

*Xavier Chevalier, Florent Eymard, and Yves Henrotin*

Osteoarthritis (OA) is the most common form of articular disease, involving 27 millions of people in the United States, and is one of the major causes of disability in the elderly [9].

OA process involved all the structures of the joint and is marked by cartilage destruction, synovial membrane inflammation, subchondral bone remodeling, and meniscal and ligament injuries.

The Osteoarthritis Research Society International (OARSI) committee has worked to standardize biomarker investigation by advocating the use of the BIPED criteria:

- Burden of the disease—disease severity in an individual
- Investigative results—insufficient evidence to classify promising candidates in one of the other categories
- Prognosis—predicting the incidence or progression of the disease
- Efficacy of intervention—indicative of treatment efficacy
- Diagnosis—distinguishing the presence or the absence of disease

These are the categories in which biomarkers can be applied to clinical use [19]. A sixth category was later added—safety—which involves identifying adverse effects and providing means of safety [19].

Among these categories, diagnosis and prognosis, including the prediction of treatment response, are particularly relevant to improving the clinical management of patients with knee or hip OA. Diagnosis biomarker may ideally identify patients in early stage of the disease where treatment may be the most effective.

Several biochemical markers have been studied for years as diagnostic and/or prognostic biomarkers [13, 14, 16, 18], although there is no consensus of any validated biomarker for incidence or progression of the disease (knee or hip OA) that can be implemented in our daily practice [13].

In this review, we will focus on the most promising *old* biomarker for the incidence and the progression of knee and hip OA (excluding hand OA) and give perspective on new biomarkers for the future. Synovial fluid biomarkers as well as markers from hand OA that represent very specific problems have been excluded from this review.

## LIMITATIONS IN THE INTERPRETATION OF SERUM BIOMARKERS

Several limitations exist in interpreting the diagnostic or the prognostic value of serum level of biomarker. Recent review published in the official journal of the OARSI summarizes the good practice for the trials on biomarkers [11].

In one hand, some limitations are related to the dosage itself and the type of assay, and, in the other hand, to the environmental condition like food intake, physical activity, and circadian rhythm. All these conditions must be verified before the use of a dosage in clinical study. The techniques should be reproducible and internationally validated by several laboratories, the coefficient of variations of the dosage should at best not exceed 10%, and the value should be referred to several confounding factors such as age, sex, body mass index (BMI), clinical phase, as well as bone status concerning marker of bone turnover.

The type of population (old, middle age, young), the phenotype of the disease, and the burden of the disease, which may increase with aging, should also be taken into account when interpreting the value of any biomarker assumed to reflect the evolution of one single OA joint.

On the other hand, discrepancy in the literature may also result from difference in the outcome definition for incidence and progression of knee or hip OA [13, 16]. Otherwise, the design of the study, the optimization of the data, and the duration of the follow-up may all contribute to the lack of reproducible results in the literature [13, 16].

One very important point to consider in terms of prognostic value of any biomarker is the dynamic variations of the serum level overtime. One study by Sharif et al. [17] has shown that serum level of cartilage oligomeric protein (COMP) is dynamic and more reflects the upcoming variations of joint-space narrowing rather than the long-term evolution over years. However, the problem might be complicated by the nonlinear relationship between biomarkers and some structural parameters. A biomarker reflects a metabolic change that is not necessarily related to structural or clinical changes. Henceforth, one may question the relevance to qualify a biomarker on the basis of its relationship with clinical and radiological criteria. A soluble biomarker primarily investigates a change in the metabolism of a tissue and an organ, and not a structural change that may result from one-time trauma.

At the end of the day, some of biomarkers have a diagnostic or a prognostic value for knee or hip OA compared with healthy subjects, despite the presence of an important overlap between groups, making the definition of a cut off value very difficult [13, 14, 16, 18].

## THE MOST INVESTIGATED BIOMARKERS: URINARY CTX-II AND SERUM COMP

### uCTX-II: Biomarker of Cartilage and Bone Remodeling

Urinary carboxy-terminal telopeptide of collagen type II (uCTX-II) is the biomarker that has been the most studied. It was discovered as a marker of type II collagen degradation [13, 16].

Data from the CHECK (Cohort Hip and Cohort Knee followed up to 5 years, including 1002 patients with early-stage symptomatic knee and/or hip OA) suggested release of CTX-II epitope from bone [3]. Actually, uCTX-II level was more strongly associated with the bone degradation markers than with the bone synthesis marker (sPIIANP) or with other cartilage markers (s845, sCOMP) [3]. Furthermore, it has been found that uCTX-II to be primarily derived from osteoclast resorption of calcified cartilage, and the localization epitope occurs at the bone–cartilage interface [1].

This lack of tissue specificity is supported by the strong sensibility of this biomarker to bone antiresorptive drugs, such as bisphosphonate and strontium ranelate.

Thus, uCTX-II is now regarded as marker of cartilage and bone remodeling, expressing the status of the borderline region between bone and cartilage. This lack of specificity makes the interpretation of CTX-II very difficult.

## Diagnostic Value in Knee OA and Hip OA

Recent literature review and meta-analysis clearly indicate that uCTX-II is one of the best markers of the incidence and of the progression of both knee and hip OA [13, 16]. Pooling different cohorts (the GARP, twin study in UK, Rotterdam study, Chingford study), it has been demonstrated that the higher levels of uCTX-II are related to higher risk of incident knee OA and a ×4 risk factor of incident hip OA [18] in population including selected people with a high risk of developing OA.

In knee OA, uCTX-II levels were more correlated with osteophytes than with joint-space narrowing [13, 18]. Furthermore, data have shown that uCTX-II levels are more elevated in the presence of pain compared to subjects with same grade of K-L but without pain.

## Burden of the Disease

In knee OA, uCTX-II may be a sensitive marker for the severity of the disease [18].

### Progression

In a recent review, most of the studies (seven positive and only one negative) show that uCTX-II is a prognostic risk factor of progression in knee OA [16]. One of the best studies is the Rotterdam study including 1235 participants, in which uCTX-II levels in the highest quartile were at six times higher risk for knee OA progression [in 13, 16].

Similarly, uCTX-II has shown the capacity to predict cartilage loss measured on MRI over 21 months by a risk ratio of 10 [13, 16].

In hip OA, except the Rotterdam study (in which the highest quartile were at eight times higher risk for hip OA progression), the value of uCTX-II as a prognostic factor is weak in terms of OR [14].

However, those results are still controversial.

## COMP: Biomarker of Matrix Production and Differentiation

The second main biomarker is the level of COMP. In the serum, COMP is a mechanosensitive molecule present in cartilage matrix. Data from the literature concerning the diagnostic and the prognostic value of serum COMP (sCOMP) are sufficiently large to draw robust conclusions.

### Diagnostic Value

Four studies show an increased risk for the incidence of knee and hip OA [4]. In a large scale meta-analysis, sCOMP was associated with the prevalence and the incidence of knee OA (Relative Risk: 3.25) [18]. However, sCOMP was not associated with the severity of the knee OA, while uCTX-II was [18].

In hip OA, sCOMP demonstrated a high diagnostic value for the incidence. It was weakly associated with the presence except in patients with more severe disease (1.3–2.89 times more elevated) than those with less severe disease [14].

### Burden of the Disease

sCOMP level in a large cohort of women with hand OA correlates with the number of joints affected by OA but was negatively correlated with the IP joints with joint-space narrowing (JSN) [13, 16].

### Prognosis

In knee OA, sCOMP demonstrates a positive value in the Valdes and in the Sharif studies [17, 18]. It was nonconclusive in others studies [16].

Baseline sCOMP level seems to have a moderate prognostic value for the progression on knee OA defined after 5 years as a progression over 2 mm of JSN or total knee replacement (TKR) [17]. Most interesting was the observation that an increase of sCOMP (measured at baseline, 2 and 5 years) precedes the immediate progression of the disease [17].

But, changes between sCOMP level and progression of knee OA may be more subtle.

Interestingly, the sCOMP levels recorded 5 hours of physical activity, (30 minutes walking) were negatively associated with cartilage thickness in the total femur and tibial cartilage at 5 years of follow-up, suggesting that exercise may be associated with abnormal tissue metabolism [4].

For hip OA, three studies reported elevations of sCOMP associated with progression of hip OA but with a very small effect size [5].

### Deamidated Form of COMP

As extracellular proteins aged, they undergo and accumulate nonenzymatic post-translational modifications such as deamination that cannot be repaired. In an analysis of 450 participants from the Johnston County Osteoarthritis Project controlled for age, gender, and race, D-COMP was associated with radiographic hip but not with knee OA severity [2].

## Lesson from the CHECK Cohort

The CHECK gives a good example of how it is difficult to compare studies between them, especially comparing early and late stage of disease. For example, the CHECK is a cohort study of early-stage symptomatic knee and/or hip OA. Progression and incidence were based on K-L definition. Several biomarkers have been obtained at baseline ($n = 801$) and 5-year follow-up ($n = 723$).

This cohort raises some unexpected results [20]. Thus, uCTX-II and sCOMP were negatively associated with the incidence of knee OA; this negative association was found especially in patients with low bone turnover. On the contrary, both uCTX-II and sCOMP were positively associated with incident radiographic hip OA, an association that holds true only in painful hip OA [20]. Again, this underlines the difficulty to interpret data of unspecific biomarker, confounded by the metabolism of other connective tissue, and the difficulty to use these biomarkers in the general population in which OA patients may present comorbidities or abnormalities in bone remodeling.

In terms of progression, both sCOMP and uCTX-II were associated with knee OA progression, while for hip OA only CS846 epitope was associated with the progression of painful hips [20]. Otherwise, bone turnover shows inconsistent associations with radiographic knee and hip OA [20]. This means that some biomarkers are more predictive of the symptoms progression than with structural changes.

### Other Markers of Collagen Degradation

C2M is marker of collagen degradation that reflects degradation by MMPs (serum MP-degraded collagen type II), and C2C is another epitope recognized after collagen type II cleavage associated with knee OA incidence and progression [13, 16, 18]. The most innovative studies concern the collagen-degraded product called the Coll2-1, which seems to be specific to collagen type II degradation [6]. This fragment could be nitrosylated: the Coll2-1$NO_2$ as the consequence of a secondary transformation by oxidation of the collagen fragments [6]. Both fragments were found to be localized in the cartilage matrix in OA tissue [6] (Figs. 5-1 and 5-2).

## BIOMARKERS OF BONE TURNOVER

In the CHECK cohort, markers of bone turnover such as type I collagen C-telopeptide (CTX-1) and N-telopeptide (NTX-1), the N-propeptide

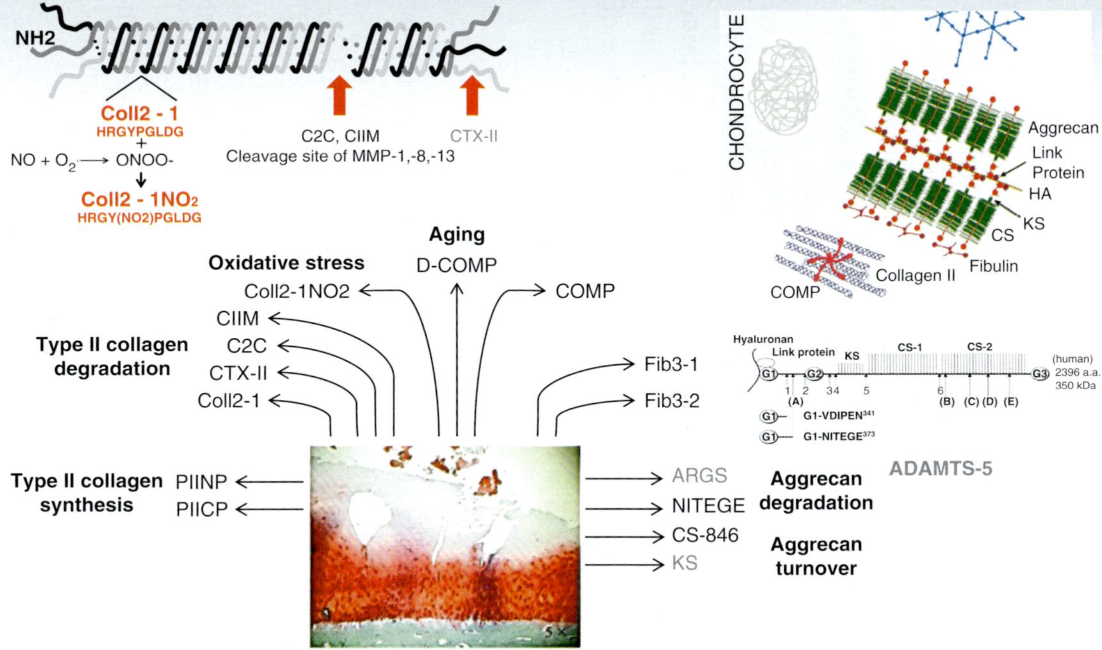


**FIGURE 5-1** Biomarkers of cartilage metabolism. Biomarker research was mainly focused on cartilage collagen, and most particularly on the type of collagen molecule that is most abundant and the most specific molecule of the cartilage. Numerous biomarkers evaluated type II collagen degradation, including Coll2-1, which is a denaturation biomarker located in triple helix, C2C, CIIM, which are neoepitope generate at collagenase cleavage site, and CTX-II, which is located at the telopeptide. PIINP and PIICP are biomarkers of type II collagen synthesis. Other post-transcriptionally modified epitopes reflect more the oxidative stress like Coll2-1$NO_2$, which is the nitrated form of Coll2-1, and D-COMP deamidated, which is the deaminated form of COMP, a process occurring during ageing. Fib3-1 and Fib3-2 are fragments of fibulin-3, a matrix protein-binding aggrecan, and are involved in the control of chondrocyte hypertrophy. Finally, aggrecan degradation is investigated by measuring body fluid neoepitope like ARGS generated by ADAMTS-5. This means that we have a well-stocked tool box to monitor cartilage metabolism. ADAMTS-5, a disintegrin and metalloproteinase with thrombospondin motifs -5.

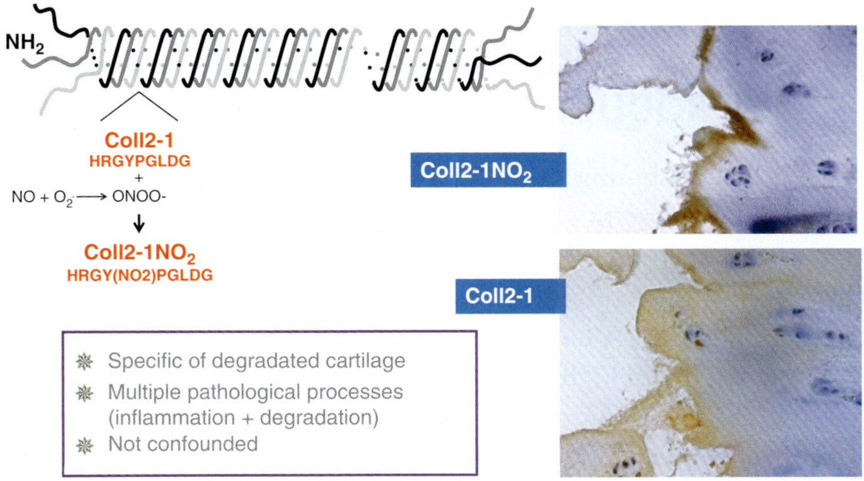


**FIGURE 5-2** Coll2-1 and Coll2-1$NO_2$ are two cartilage-specific biomarkers. Coll2-1 is denaturated epitope located in the triple helical part of the type II collagen molecule. This peptide contains one tyrosine, which is sensitive to nitration during oxidative stress. For this reason, we have developed an immunoassay that specifically measures Coll2-1$NO_2$ as an indicator of the oxidative-related cartilage degradation. As you can observe on these immuhistochemical pictures, Coll2-1 and Coll2-1$NO_2$ epitopes are expressed only in the superficial layer of cartilage lesion.

(PINP), and osteocalcin were associated with the presence of knee OA but not with incident or the progression. As opposed to findings in knee OA, there was a negative association of bone marker levels with presence and progression of radiographic hip OA [20]. Though, there are numbers of reports showing that markers of bone turnover in knee OA also indicate the progression of the disease [18].

One isoform of the C-telopeptide α1 chain is nonisomerized and is mostly found in newly formed bone. In the prediction of the OA progression cohort, uαCTX-I was not associated with knee OA severity but was associated with changes reflecting radiographic progression over 3 years, while on the other hand, uCTX-II reflected the severity at baseline but was only related to progression of osteophytes [8].

## COMBINATION BIOMARKER OF MATRIX DEGRADATION AND MATRIX PRODUCTION

At best, combining local (SF) and systemic biomarker assessment may help. More than 10 years ago, Garnero et al. (referred in a recent review by Lotz et al [13]) conducted several studies in knee and hip OA, showing that the best predictor of knee OA progression was the combination of a low level of PIIANP (a marker of type collagen synthesis) and a high level of uCTX-II. At 1 year of evolution of knee OA, the relative risk of progression on JSN is much higher when combining uCTX-II and PIIANP, another marker of collagen synthesis (RR: 4–6), than taking one solely (RR: 2.7 and 2.9) [13].

## BIOMARKERS OF INFLAMMATION

### C-Reactive Protein

Ultra sensible C-reactive protein (CRP) has been shown to increase in several of OA phenotypes, notably in erosive hand OA and in rapid destructive hip OA where its level is elevated compared with standard OA [10].

A recent meta-analysis has included 32 studies in respecting an acceptable methodology.

Among 17 studies comparing the serum level of usCRP in patients with knee or hip OA (2354 patients) and in subjects without OA (3118), CRP levels were weakly elevated with OA in most of the studies but with a nonsignificant mean difference of 1.19 (0.64–1.73), leading to inconclusive association [10]. Levels were significantly associated with pain and decreased physical function.

No significant associations were found between us-CRP levels and the progression even if there was a trend for a predictive value of us-CRP. However, this concerns studies with small number of patients (between 23 and 30) [10].

## Hyaluronic Acid

Hyaluronic acid (HA) serum level correlates with the number of joints affected by osteophytes but not with JSN [13, 16]. There was a weak correlation between acid hyaluronic serum level and the severity of knee OA [13, 16].

In a 5-year follow-up study, the baseline level of HA was higher in the group of progressors (more than 2 mm) (72.7 ng/mL) compared with the nonprogressors (46.3 ng/mL) [17]. In the Echodia study, 3 years' study in hip OA comparing diacerein with placebo, a level of HA superior to 137 μg/L, was predictive of progression in placebo group [13].

## Adipokines

Adipokines are secreted by the adipose tissue but also in the joint. Adipokines may indirectly reflect the systemic participation of the adipose tissue in OA.

Four major adipokines have been studied in OA: leptin, adiponectin, vifstatin, and resistin. Their actions on cartilage and subchondral bone are complex and somewhat contradictory.

Serum levels of leptin, adiponectin, and resistin are sex dependent (more elevated in women than in men), and serum levels of leptin and vifstatin are positively correlated with BMI while the serum level of adiponectin is lower in obese people [15]. In the CHECK cohort, only the serum level of resistin showed positive association with presence and incidence of radiographic knee OA (especially in the subgroup where adiponectin levels were higher) that were largely independent of BMI [20]. However, today no conclusion could be drawn concerning the diagnostic and the prognostic values of any adipokines [15].

# PREARTHRITIC CONDITIONS: AN EARLY STAGE OF OSTEOARTHRITS

Another way to validate the diagnostic value of a biomarker is to look to preosteoarthritic conditions. The Swedish team led by Lohmander has done tremendous works in patients with recent posttraumatic injuries of the knee. Those patients have been followed up for as long as 10 years. To summarize, after a traumatic knee injury, they show a long-term (over years) turnover of matrix components not only from cartilage such as fragments of proteoglycans, tenascin, and collagen type II fragment (C2C) but also from cartilage bone interface such as the bone sialin protein, together with long-term production of cytokines, which are released in the synovial fluid (SF) [12]. Those abnormal turnover might be the consequence of a low-grade synovitis, and in fine results in an increase in the degradative process [12], though this increase may also indicate an increased synthesis within the joint [12].

## MARKERS OF THE EFFICACY OF INTERVENTION

Though there are numbers of studies linking the efficacy of a potential chondroprotective drugs and levels of several biomarkers, none has been clearly validated as the good candidate. This limitation is mainly due to the lack of any approved so-called DMARD in OA [13].

Henrotin et al. [5] reported a decrease (compared with baseline level) in the urine levels of CTX-II, Coll2-1, and Coll2-1$NO_2$ at 3 months after a series of three injections of hylan GF-20, suggesting a potential chondroprotective effect of a high molecular weight HA.

## CANDIDATES FOR NOVEL BIOMARKERS IN OA: INVESTIGATIVE BIOMARKERS

The *omics* approach is a general approach which consists to measure huge number of molecules or genes expression trying to differentiate those which are present in a specific disease from healthy controls. This omics approach includes genomics (beyond the scope of this review), proteomics, lipidomics, metabolomics, and transcriptomics.

Different patterns of proteins have been studied in OA using different approaches. In the body fluid, serum SF, and serum, the collection is much easier, but needs an affinity depletion to remove the most abundant molecules that mask the signal of other less abundant molecules. For example, synovial fluid contains abundant serum proteins and highly anionic hyaluronan that contribute to the difficulty in analyzing this fluid.

A recent literature review highlights the progress done in this field [7]. Four candidate's biomarkers, a glycosylated peptide from hemopexine, a glycosylated peptide from $\alpha$1 acid glycoprotein, and two molecules clusterin and macrophage-stimulating protein, have been associated with knee OA [7]. Among them, the glycosylated peptide from hemopexin molecule was strongly expressed in progressors, and may suggest that glycosylation may increase during the progression of the disease [7].

Henrotin and colleagues explored new candidates' markers using a proteomic analysis from urine samples. Thirteen proteins were identified in patients with OA compared with controls. Among them, fibulin3-1 and fibulin3-2 fragments were of particular interest. The serum levels of these two new biomarkers were found to be elevated in patients with OA compared with healthy subjects [7].

Metabolomic is another promising approach, which may allow emerging new kind of serological markers. However, the number of testable metabolites could be very high (up to thousands), and the interpretation of variation between OA population and non-OA should also take into account any comorbidities such diabetes and metabolic syndrome.

Serum metabolites profile, such as decreased histidine and glycine levels, might help to discriminate patients with knee OA and healthy controls.

## CONCLUSIONS

Actually, none of the current biomarker exhibit sufficient power to discriminate incident OA, progression of the hip or knee OA, burden of OA, and being sensitive to change under a cartilage protective therapy. Two biomarkers, uCTX-II and sCOMP, appear to be the most robust biomarkers, even if they could not be used in daily practice because they are not specific for the disease.

Certainly, we should differentiate marker of the incidence, of the preradiographic OA, of definite OA, and of progression.

In the future, we may use a combination of biomarkers (originating from different tissues such as cartilage, synovial membrane, subchondral bone) to predict the emergence and/or the progression of the disease, as well as the addition of biochemical markers plus imaging marker such as MRI for early detection of OA and for the progression.

This may rise to aggregate scores combining panel biomarkers, reflecting the metabolic changes in different disease-affected connective tissues. Combining systemic to local biomarker is an important target, despite the difficulty to assess markers into the SF in daily practice.

Another consideration is the recognition of OA phenotypes. Not all phenotypes of OA may correspond to the same biomarker.

Finally, beside the clinical and imaging features, soluble biomarkers should be considered to evaluate the response of patient to treatment. Metabolic changes in joint tissue may occur early in OA development, before the appearance of symptoms and structural changes, and should be considered a therapeutic outcome.

This target is one of the most challenging one for the upcoming years. It may impact not only your daily practice, but also the cost of the disease in targeting responders for a treatment.

## REFERENCES

1. Bay-Jensen AC, Andersen TL, Charni-Ben Tabassi N, Kristensen PW, Kjaersgaard-Andersen P, Sandell L, Garnero P, Delaissé JM. Biochemical markers of type II collagen breakdown and synthesis are positioned at specific sites in human osteoarthritic knee cartilage. Osteoarthritis Cartilage 2008;16:615–23.
2. Catterall JB, Hsueh MF, Stabler TV, McCudden CR, Bolognesi M, Zura R, Jordan JM, Renner JB, Feng S, Kraus VB. Protein modification by deamidation indicates variations in joint extracellular matrix turnover. J Biol Chem 2012;287:4640–51.
3. de Klerk B, Lafeber FP, van Spil WE. Associations of CTX-II with biochemical markers of bone turnover raise questions about its tissue origin: new insights from CHECK. Ann Rheum Dis 2014;73:e39.
4. Erhart-Hledik JC, Favre J, Asay JL, Smith RL, Giori NJ, Mündermann A, Andriacchi TP. A relationship between mechanically-induced changes in serum

cartilage oligomeric matrix protein (COMP) and changes in cartilage thickness after 5 years. Osteoarthritis Cartilage 2012;20:1309–15.

5. Henrotin Y, Chevalier X, Deberg M, Balblanc JC, Richette P, Mulleman D, Maillet B, Rannou F, Piroth C, Mathieu P, Conrozier T; Osteoarthritis Group of French Society of Rheumatology. Early decrease of serum biomarkers of type II collagen degradation (Coll2-1) and joint inflammation (Coll2-1 NO2) by hyaluronic acid intra-articular injections in patients with knee osteoarthritis: a research study part of the Biovisco study. J Orthop Res 2013;31:901–7.
6. Henrotin Y, Deberg M, Mathy-Hartert M, Deby-Dupont G. Biochemical biomarkers of oxidative collagen damage. Adv Clin Chem 2009;49:31–55.
7. Hsueh MF, Önnerfjord P, Kraus VB. Biomarkers and proteomic analysis of osteoarthritis. Matrix Biol 2014;39:56–66.
8. Huebner JL, Bay-Jensen AC, Huffman KM, He Y, Leeming DJ, McDaniel GE, Karsdal MA, Kraus VB. Alpha C-telopeptide of type I collagen is associated with subchondral bone turnover and predicts progression of joint space narrowing and osteophytes in osteoarthritis. Arthritis Rheumatol 2014;66:2440–9.
9. Issa SN, Sharma L. Epidemiology of osteoarthritis: an update. Curr Rheumatol Rep 2006;8:7–15.
10. Jin X, Beguerie JR, Zhang W, Blizzard L, Otahal P, Jones G, Ding C. Circulating C reactive protein in osteoarthritis: a systematic review and meta-analysis. Ann Rheum Dis 2015;74:703–10.
11. Kraus VB, Blanco FJ, Englund M, Henrotin Y, Lohmander LS, Losina E, Önnerfjord P, Persiani S. OARSI Clinical Trials Recommendations: soluble biomarker assessments in clinical trials in osteoarthritis. Osteoarthritis Cartilage 2015;23:686–97.
12. Kumahashi N, Swärd P, Larsson S, Lohmander LS, Frobell R, Struglics A. Type II collagen C2C epitope in human synovial fluid and serum after knee injury: associations with molecular and structural markers of injury. Osteoarthritis Cartilage 2015;23:1506–12.
13. Lotz M, Martel Pelletier J, Christiansen C, Brandi ML, Bruyére O, Chapurlat R, Collette J, Cooper C, Giacovelli G, Kanis JA, et al. Value of biomarkers in osteoarthritis: current status and perspectives. Ann Rheum Dis 2013;72:1756–63.
14. Nepple JJ, Thomason KM, An TW, Harris-Hayes M, Clohisy JC. What is the utility of biomarkers for assessing the pathophysiology of hip osteoarthritis? A systematic review. Clin Orthop Relat Res 2015;473:1683–701.
15. Poonpet T, Honsawek S. Adipokines: Biomarkers for osteoarthritis? World J Orthop 2014;5:319–2.
16. Saberi HF, Runhaar J, van Meurs JB, Bierma-Zeinstra SM. Biomarkers for osteoarthritis: Can they be used for risk assessment? A systematic review. Maturitas 2015;82:36–49.
17. Sharif M, Kirwan JR, Elson CJ, Granell R, Clarke S. Suggestion of non linear or phasic progression of knee osteoarthritis based on measurements of serum cartilage oligomeric matrix protein levels over five years. Arthritis Rheum 2004;50:2479–88.

18. Valdes AM, Meulenbelt I, Chassaing E, Arden NK, Bierma-Zeinstra S, Hart D, Hofman A, Karsdal M, Kloppenburg M, Kroon HM, et al. Large scale meta-analysis of urinary C-terminal telopeptide, serum cartilage oligomeric protein and matrix metalloprotease degraded type II collagen and their role in prevalence, incidence and progression of osteoarthritis. Osteoarthritis Cartilage 2014;22(5):683–89.
19. Van Spil WE, De Groot A, Lemzs WF, Oostveen JC, Lafeber FP. Serum and urinary biochemical markers for knee and hip osteoarthritis: a systematic review applying the consensus BIPED criteria. Osteoarthritis Cartilage 2010;18:605–12.
20. Van Spil WE, Welsing PM, Bierma-Zeinstra SM, Bijlsma JW, Roorda LD, Cats HA, Lafeber FP. The ability of systemic biochemical markers to reflect presence, incidence, and progression of early-stage radiographic knee and hip osteoarthritis: data from CHECK. Osteoarthritis Cartilage 2015;23:1388–97.

CHAPTER 6

# Joint Imaging in Osteoarthritis: What Are the Readouts and How Are They Related to Pain?

*Frank W. Roemer and Ali Guermazi*

Osteoarthritis (OA) is the most common form of arthritis and a leading cause of disability worldwide, largely because of pain, the primary symptom of the disease. Approximately 10–12% of the adult population have symptomatic OA, and recent estimates suggest that 250 million people worldwide are burdened by the presence of knee OA [4].

OA is a heterogeneous disease that is characterized structurally by progressive cartilage loss, subchondral bone remodeling, osteophyte formation, and synovial inflammation with resultant joint pain and increasing functional disability. However, while pain and disability are frequent complaints of patients with symptomatic OA, approximately 50% of persons with structural changes consistent with OA are asymptomatic [11].

Despite articular cartilage being one of the hallmark features of OA, cartilage is an aneural tissue, and we still do not have a clear understanding of how the various structural changes of other joint tissues interact and how they account for the development and persistence of pain. Similarly, the variance of pain explained by independent structural changes or their cumulative effect and their interactions remain poorly understood.

Imaging is essential for assessing structural joint damage and disease progression in OA. Conventional radiography is still the basis for diagnosis and is the most commonly used imaging modality, while magnetic resonance imaging (MRI) is widely applied in epidemiologic studies and clinical trials with limited indications in a routine clinical setting. MRI provides an ideal noninvasive means to investigate OA pathogenesis and pathophysiology. Baseline and longitudinal differences in morphology and composition of various joint tissues can be used to both measure and predict disease progression as well as clinical correlates and outcomes including pain, potentially providing early indicators or biomarkers of disease. A number of quantitative and qualitative MRI features such as bone marrow lesions (BMLs), synovitis, and subchondral bone attrition have already been identified that may be associated with OA disease progression, and more biomarkers will undoubtedly be identified as more long-term data become available.

Further, imaging will play an increasing role in the evaluation of patients with osteoarthritic joint pain particularly during the developmental process of novel therapeutic approaches such as the anti-nerve growth factor (a-NGF) compounds that have shown good analgesic efficacy and improvement in function in patients with OA. However, despite initial promising data, a-NGF trials in OA had been suspended for years because of concerns over accelerated rates of OA progression and other complications such as subchondral insufficiency fracture and osteonecrosis. Since a-NGF therapies offer potential as the first new class of analgesics for many years, future studies assessing a-NGF compounds will have to include stringent eligibility criteria and will require rigorous safety monitoring. While disease-modifying structural effects are not expected in a-NGF treatment, imaging plays a crucial role in clinical trials to define eligibility of potential participants with focus on exclusion criteria and to monitor safety during the course of these studies to either identify subjects at risk for fast OA progression prior inclusion or withdraw subjects from study early to avoid adverse events such as rapid progressive OA [18].

A detailed discussion of the different tissues within the joint and their respective contribution to symptoms are discussed in the following. While it is recognized that increased neuronal activity from the periphery (i.e., peripheral sensitization) may contribute to plasticity changes in the central nervous system (i.e., central sensitization, structural anatomic correlates involved in the complex nociceptive pathways including the peripheral nerves), the spinal cord or brain structures are not discussed.

## RADIOGRAPHIC FINDINGS AND PAIN

Radiography is the simplest, least expensive, and most widely available imaging technique. It enables detection of bony features associated with OA, including marginal osteophytes, subchondral sclerosis, attrition, and subchondral cysts (Fig. 6-1) [1]. The presence of these features can be observed in any joint that is affected by OA. In addition to subjective assessment of joint-space narrowing (JSN), radiography allows quantitative measurement of joint space width (JSW), an indirect surrogate of cartilage thickness and meniscal integrity, although precise and direct assessment of each of these particular structures is not possible with radiography. Nevertheless, progression of JSN is the most commonly used endpoint for the assessment of OA progression, and complete loss of JSW characterized by bone-on-bone contact indicates so-called end-stage OA, which is considered one of the indications for joint replacement.

The severity of OA can be estimated using semiquantitative scoring systems. Published atlases provide image examples that represent specific grades [1]. The Kellgren and Lawrence (KL) scale [15] is a widely accepted scheme used for defining the presence or absence of radiographic OA, using grade 2 disease as the threshold for the presence of radiographic OA. The KL scheme is a composite measure comprising the presence or absence of marginal osteophytes and JSN. Patients with clinical signs and symptoms of OA with a KL grade of 0 or 1 may fulfill the clinical criteria of OA but will be considered having preradiographic OA from a structural view point. A modified, simplified version of the KL grading scheme is summarized in Table 6-1. Recently, a modification of KL grading was suggested to improve the sensitivity to change in longitudinal knee OA studies, including the addition of JSN to the radiographic diagnosis of knee OA [9].

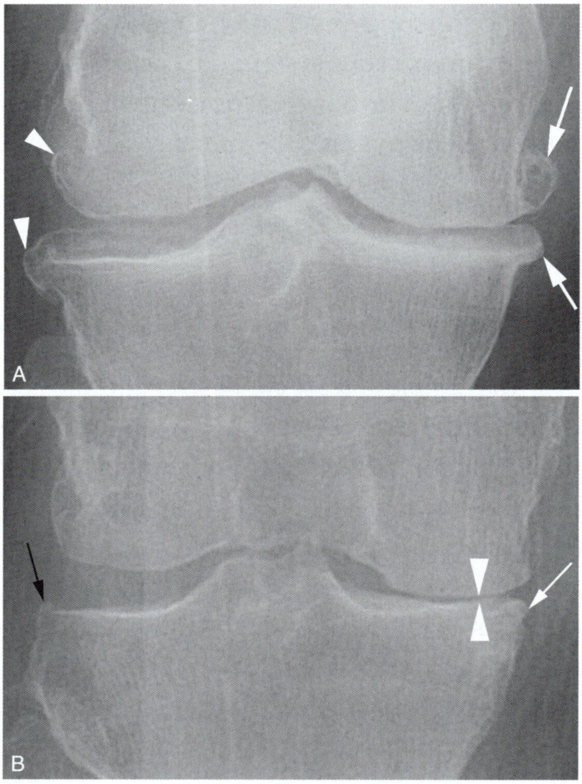


**FIGURE 6-1** Radiographic manifestations of osteoarthritis. **A:** AP radiograph of the knee shows large marginal osteophytes of the medial (*arrows*) and lateral (*arrowheads*) tibiofemoral compartments. Note additional joint-space narrowing of the medial compartment. Image represents the hypertrophic phenotype of tibiofemoral osteoarthritis with severe osteophyte formation and comparatively discrete joint-space narrowing. **B:** Atrophic phenotype of osteoarthritis. AP radiograph of the knee shows severe joint-space narrowing of the medial compartment (*arrowheads*). Only tiny osteophytes are seen at the medial (*white arrow*) and lateral (*black arrow*) joint margins.

The Osteoarthritis Research Society International (OARSI) Atlas [1] takes a different approach and grades tibiofemoral JSN and osteophytes separately for each compartment of the knee, all on a scale of 0–3 (Table 6-2). In contrast to the KL scheme, the OARSI Atlas does not give the grades definitions but displays specific image examples to illustrate the different grades for each compartment. This compartmental scoring appears to be more sensitive to longitudinal radiographic

TABLE 6-1 **Description of Kellgren and Lawrence and Modified Kellgren and Lawrence Grading Systems for Knee OA**

| | Original Kellgren and Lawrence Classification | Modified Kellgren and Lawrence Classification | Radiographic Osteoarthritis |
|---|---|---|---|
| Grade 0 | No feature of osteoarthritis | No feature of osteoarthritis | No |
| Grade 1 | Doubtful joint-space narrowing and possible osteophytic lipping | Equivocal osteophyte | No |
| Grade 2 | Definite osteophytes and possible joint-space narrowing | Unequivocal osteophyte | Yes |
| Grade 3 | Moderate multiple osteophytes, definite joint-space narrowing, and some sclerosis and possible deformity of bone ends | Joint-space narrowing | Yes |
| Grade 4 | Large osteophytes, marked joint-space narrowing, severe sclerosis, and definite deformity of bone ends | Bone-to-bone appearance | Yes |

*Source*: Adapted from Guermazi A, Hunter DJ, Roemer FW. Plain radiography and magnetic resonance imaging diagnostics in osteoarthritis: validated staging and scoring. J Bone Joint Surg Am 2009;91:54–62.

TABLE 6-2 **Osteoarthritis Research Society International (OARSI) Grading System for Knee OA Features**

| Feature | Grade |
|---|---|
| Medial femoral osteophyte | 0–3 |
| Medial tibial osteophyte | 0–3 |
| Lateral femoral osteophyte | 0–3 |
| Lateral tibial osteophyte | 0–3 |
| Medial tibiofemoral joint-space narrowing | 0–3 |
| Lateral tibiofemoral joint-space narrowing | 0–3 |

*Source*: For corresponding images see Altman RD, Gold GE. Atlas of individual radiographic features in osteoarthritis, revised. Osteoarthritis Cartilage 2007;15:A1–56. Accessed at: http://dx.doi.org/10.1016/j.joca.2006.11.009.

changes than KL grading. Note that semiquantitative scoring is applied not only to the knee joint, but also to other joints, particularly the hip and the interphalangeal joints of the hands.

In population-based studies, a significant discordance between radiographically diagnosed OA and knee pain has been reported. While radiographic evidence of joint damage predisposes to joint pain, the underlying pathologies leading to pain cannot be readily discerned from radiography alone and may require consideration of other factors. Novel study designs are one approach to deal with the so-called structure–symptom discordance. For example, when interindividual differences influencing the pain experience, including genetics, sensitization, mood, coping, catastrophizing, and the social context, among others, are adequately accounted for, a strong relationship between radiographic OA and knee pain was observed [17]. Using a within-person knee-matched approach to control for such between-person differences, radiographic severity has been demonstrated to have a strong dose response relationship with presence of pain, pain severity, and incident pain [17]. Despite radiography being the most widely used first-line imaging modality for structural OA evaluation, its inherent limitations should be noted, including lack of ability to directly visualize most of OA-related pathological features in and around the joint that are potentially responsible to explain symptoms related with the disease, lack of sensitivity to longitudinal change, missing specificity of JSN, and technical difficulties regarding reproducibility of positioning of the joints in longitudinal studies.

## MAGNETIC RESONANCE IMAGING IN OSTEOARTHRITIS

Because of high cost per examination, MRI is not routinely used in the clinical initial assessment or during disease follow-up of OA patients. However, MRI has become a key imaging tool for OA research thanks to its ability to visualize pathologies that are not detected on radiographs (i.e., articular cartilage, menisci, ligaments, synovium, capsular structures, fluid collections, and BMLs). MRI offers several advantages over radiography: The joint can be evaluated, including all relevant tissues involved in the disease process; multiple tissue changes can be monitored simultaneously over several time points; pathologic changes of preradiographic OA can be detected at a much earlier stage of the disease; and early compositional changes within joint tissues (e.g., cartilage and menisci) can be assessed before morphologic changes become apparent.

MRI may be evaluated by semiquantitative scoring approaches, by 3D segmentation, or using compositional techniques. Several MRI scoring systems are available for the assessment of OA, with each having advantages and disadvantages. For assessment of synovitis, contrast-enhanced (CE) MRI enables more accurate evaluation than scoring of nonenhanced MRI data. Cartilage or meniscus quantification requires segmentation and exploits the three-dimensional nature of MRI data sets to evaluate tissue dimensions (such as thickness, areas volume, and others) as continuous variables. So-called compositional MRI allows visualization of the biochemical properties of different joint tissues. These techniques are very sensitive to early, premorphologic changes that cannot be seen on conventional MR imaging. The role of compositional MRI for elucidating associations with pain incidence, progression, or fluctuation needs to be shown.

A detailed review article focusing on semiquantitative MRI assessment of OA has been published recently [10]. In addition to the three well-established scoring systems—the Whole Organ MRI Score (WORMS), the Knee Osteoarthritis Scoring System (KOSS), and the Boston Leeds Osteoarthritis Knee Score (BLOKS)—a new scoring system called the MRI Osteoarthritis Knee Score (MOAKS) [13] has been added to the literature. Of the three systems, WORMS and BLOKS have been widely disseminated and used, though only a limited number of studies have directly compared the two systems. Two recent studies identified the relative strengths and weaknesses of the two systems in regard to certain features assumed to be most relevant to the natural history of the disease, including cartilage, meniscus, and BMLs. Both these systems have undergone unpublished modifications that make it difficult for general readers to determine the differences between the original description and how they have been applied in later research. The use of within-grade changes for longitudinal assessment of cartilage damage and BMLs is a good example, which has also been applied to radiographic OA assessment in order to increase sensitivity to change. Within-grade scoring describes progression or improvement of a lesion that does not meet the criteria of a full-grade change but does represent a definite visual change. It has become common practice to incorporate these within-grade changes whenever longitudinal cartilage assessment is contemplated, and a recent study demonstrated that within-grade changes in semiquantitative MRI assessment of cartilage and BMLs are valid, and their use may increase the sensitivity of semiquantitative readings in detecting longitudinal changes in these structures [19].

By integrating expert readers' experience with all of the available scoring tools and the published data comparing different scoring systems, MOAKS was developed as a refined scoring tool for cross-sectional and longitudinal semiquantitative MRI assessment of knee OA. It includes semiquantitative scoring of the following pathological features: BMLs; subchondral cysts; articular cartilage; osteophytes; Hoffa synovitis and synovitis-effusion; meniscus; tendons and ligaments; and periarticular features such as cysts and bursitides. Since MOAKS is a new scoring system, it needs more data to demonstrate its validity and reliability when applied to large OA studies.

## PAIN AND MRI FINDINGS

One study applying direct unanesthetized examination of articular tissues in the human knee joint has provided some insight into particular structures that do and do not elicit pain when probed [5]. Utilizing imaging modalities such as MRI, several structural alterations such as meniscal tears, subchondral BMLs, subarticular bone attrition, synovitis, and effusion have been related to knee pain. Furthermore, changes in BMLs and inflammatory markers on MRI are associated with fluctuations in pain in patients with knee OA [20]. How much of the variance in pain is accounted for by structural change is not fully understood. One reason for this difficulty is that most studies focused on late disease stages when numerous pathologic changes are already commonly present. In fact, abnormalities on MRI are very common even in knees that are considered to be radiographically normal.

A systematic review examined the concurrent relation of MRI findings in OA to symptoms. Of these studies, just over half demonstrated a statistically significant association, indicating that studies to date have found inconsistent associations of structural features to symptoms [14]. Nonetheless, in general, large BMLs were strongly associated with knee pain, followed by synovitis and effusion, and cartilage volume and thickness. Interpretation of these relationships is challenging as it is not clear as to whether all of these associations are truly causal, or rather are markers of the severity of other structural pathology that may be contributing to the pain experience.

## Cartilage

Articular cartilage is both aneural and avascular. As such, cartilage is incapable of directly generating pain, inflammation, stiffness, or any of the symptoms that patients with OA typically describe at least early on in the disease course prior to potential neurovascular invasion that may occur in late or end-stage disease. During cartilage degradation, substances are released that are capable of inducing inflammation in the joint. Some studies have suggested a relation between cartilage morphometric measures and lesions and the symptoms of OA. In this context, it is important to note that this disease of the whole joint concurrently affects other tissues that do contain nociceptors. The studies that have demonstrated a relation of cartilage damage to pain have traditionally investigated the role of cartilage in predisposing to symptoms in isolation from other tissues, and as such cannot provide insight into the independent contribution of cartilage pathology to pain. A recent study suggested that areas of denuded cartilage are related to symptoms [3]. Again, the likely mechanism for symptom genesis is through secondary mechanisms such as altered biomechanics and subsequent increased loading to the underlying subchondral bone, vascular congestion of subchondral bone, leading to increased intraosseous pressure, or through synovitis secondary to articular cartilage damage with activation of synovial membrane nociceptors. Knees exhibiting denuded areas of cartilage are more likely to have concomitant potentially painful tissue pathology such as synovitis/effusion and BMLs.

## Bone Marrow Lesions

The osseous changes with the most supportive evidence for a role in symptom genesis are BMLs (Fig. 6-2). These biomechanically induced lesions in the bone marrow, reflecting the histologic changes of fibrosis, trabecular microfractures, and other manifestations of bone remodeling, play an integral if not pivotal role in the symptoms that emanate from knee OA and its structural progression [7]. More recently, their relation to pain severity and incident pain was also demonstrated [8]. Conflicting data are available, albeit from smaller studies with different methods, suggesting no relation of BMLs to pain; however, the balance of data would support a strong relation of BMLs to pain.

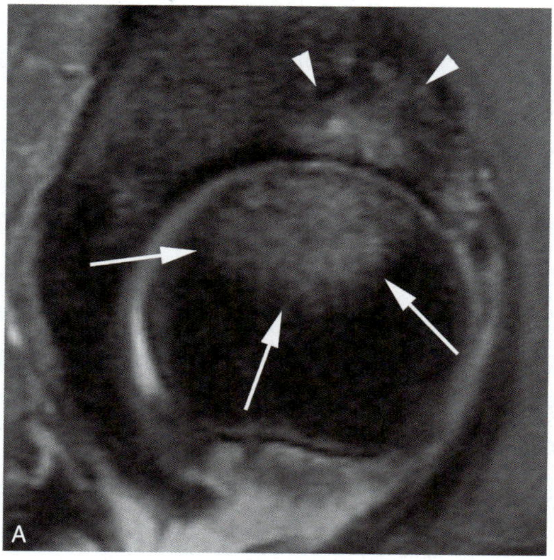


**FIGURE 6-2** Bone marrow lesions and relevance of image acquisition. **A:** Sagittal intermediate-weighted fat-suppressed MRI shows diffuse full-thickness cartilage loss at the central superior weight-bearing part of the joint. Because the cartilage is very thin, a clear delineation of acetabular and femoral cartilage is not possible. In addition, there are extensive subchondral BMLs in the femoral head (*arrows*) and acetabulum (*arrowheads*). **B:** Coronal intermediate-weighted turbo spin echo MRI shows subchondral bone marrow lesions in the medial femur (*arrows*) and tibia (*asterisk*). **C:** Corresponding coronal fast low-angle shot (FLASH) image, commonly used for cartilage segmentation, barely depicts femoral bone marrow lesion (*arrows*) and shows tibial bone marrow lesion only to a minimal extent. Note in addition marked femoral and tibial cartilage loss, marginal osteophytes, and severe meniscal extrusion.

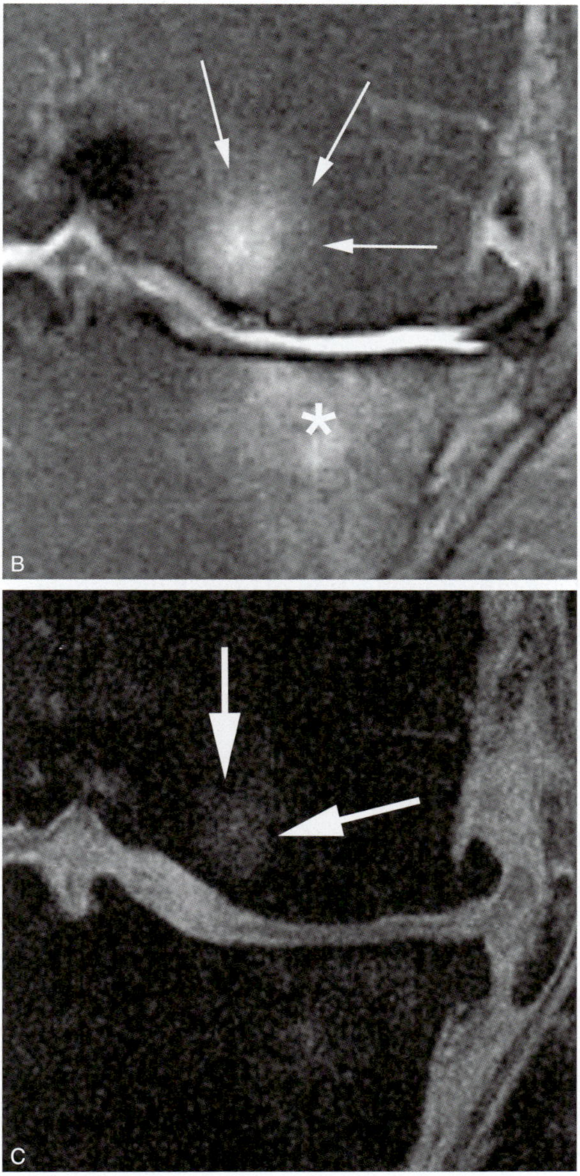


**FIGURE 6-2** *(continued)*

Other bone-related causes of pain include periostitis associated with osteophyte formation, subchondral microfractures, bone attrition, and bone angina due to decreased blood flow and elevated intraosseous pressure, which are reflected on imaging also as nonspecific

BMLs. Given the strong relationship between bony structural changes, symptoms, and structural progression, targeting these more selectively would be a major advance in delineating appropriate therapies.

## Osteophytes

One prospective cohort reported an association between increasing osteophyte size and increasing WOMAC pain severity score. In other cross-sectional analyses, osteophyte size was associated with the presence but not severity of pain [16]. In unadjusted cross-sectional analyses, osteophytes were inconsistently associated with a heterogeneous range of pain measures. In summary, osteophytes seem to be associated with longitudinally increasing pain severity and the cross-sectional presence of pain, albeit it appears unlikely that these are the actual cause of pain, but are rather a reflection of overall disease severity or are causative in regard to irritation of adjacent structures such as bursae.

## Meniscal Damage

An intact and functional meniscus is important to the preservation of joint integrity and prevention of further joint damage. In contrast, the meniscus plays a much smaller role in symptom genesis. Some emerging data that incident tears and those involving the red zone (outer rim) of the meniscus may play a limited role in symptom genesis through angiogenesis and associated sensory nerve growth exist.

The association between meniscal pathology and pain remains controversial and may reflect site-specific associations. Any meniscal damage was associated with knee pain but not after adjustment for radiographic OA [6]. Other studies reported that meniscal tears at the lateral posterior and anterior horns, but not at other sites, were significantly associated with questionnaire-assessed pain, stiffness, and function scores, or that macerated tears were associated with pain.

An unfortunate consequence of the frequent use of MRI in clinical practice is the frequent detection of meniscal tears. Degenerative lesions, described as horizontal cleavages, flap (oblique), or complex tears or meniscal maceration or destruction are associated with older age and are almost universal in persons with OA. In asymptomatic subjects with a mean age of 65 years, a tear was found in 67% using MRI, whereas in patients with symptomatic knee OA, a meniscal tear was found in 91%. Meniscal tears are nearly universal in persons with knee OA and are unlikely to be a cause of increased symptoms. The penchant to remove menisci is to be avoided, unless there are symptoms of locking or extension blockade, at which point surgical treatment often becomes necessary.

## Effusion and Synovitis

The anatomic and histologic correlates of synovial activation in OA include synovial hyperplasia, fibrosis, thickening of synovial capsule, activated synoviocytes, and in some cases, lymphocytic infiltrates (B and T cells as well as plasma cells). Synovial causes of pain include irritation of sensory nerve endings within the synovium from osteophytes and synovial inflammation that is due, at least in part, to the release of prostaglandins, leukotrienes, proteinases, neuropeptides, and cytokines. Synovitis and effusion are frequently present in OA and correlate with pain and other clinical outcomes [2, 12]. A semiquantitative measure of synovitis from the infrapatellar fat pad is associated with pain severity, and similarly, change in synovitis is associated with change in pain severity and pain fluctuation [20]. In an important caveat to this analysis, a recent study compared nonenhanced proton-density-weighted fat-suppressed (PDFS) sequences with T1-weighted (T1w) fat-suppressed (FS) contrast-enhanced sequences for semiquantitative assessment of peripatellar synovitis in OA and showed a superior association with pain for CE MRI. Fig. 6-3 shows a comparison between MRI findings of inflammation on fluid-sensitive images and T1-weighted CE images. These data suggested that signal alterations in Hoffa's fat pad on nonenhanced images do not always represent synovitis as seen on T1w CE images but are rather nonspecific albeit sensitive finding.

## Other Joint Structures and Periarticular Tissues

The relevance of other joint structures such as bursae and cysts is not fully understood. A recent study focusing on popliteal cysts and

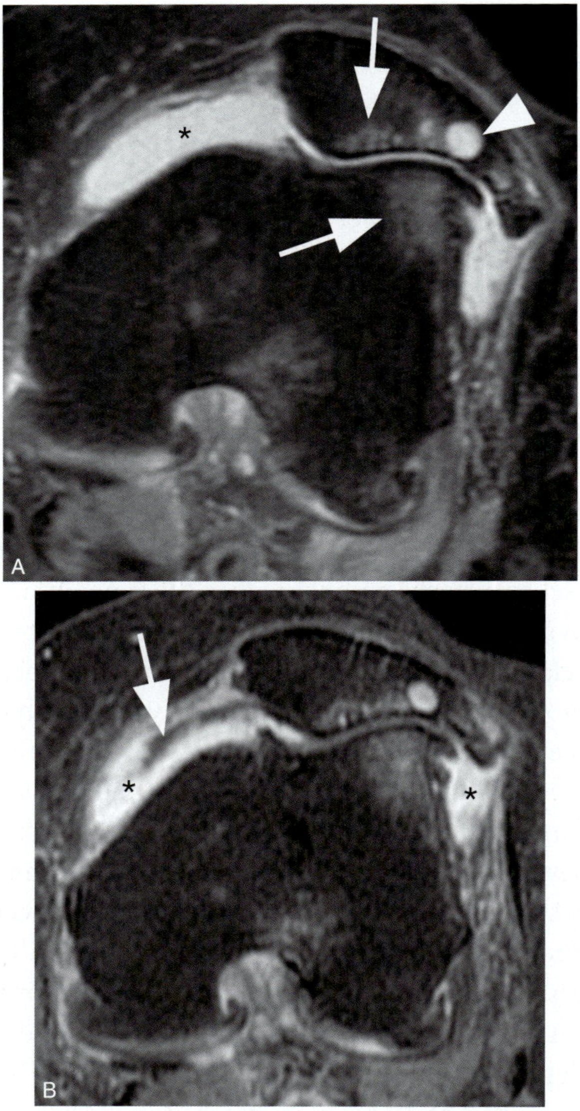


**FIGURE 6-3** Visualization of synovitis using non-contrast-enhanced and contrast-enhanced MRI. **A:** Axial proton-density-weighted fat-suppressed MRI shows marked hyperintensity within the joint cavity, suggesting severe joint effusion (*asterisk*). In addition, there is a large subchondral cyst in the lateral facet of the patella (*arrowhead*) and diffuse bone marrow edema in the lateral patella and trochlea (*arrows*). **B:** Axial T1-weighted fat-suppressed after contrast administration clearly visualizes severe synovial thickening depicted as contrast enhancement (*asterisks*). *Arrow* points to true amount of effusion, which is only discrete and visualized as linear hypointensity within the joint cavity.

subgastrocnemius bursitis reported an association with other structural damage and increased weight-bearing knee pain that become nonsignificant after adjustment for cartilage defects and BMLs. Another study focused on synovial thickening, effusion, and popliteal cysts, and did not find a difference in prevalence of popliteal cysts between subjects with and without knee pain.

## BEYOND OSTEOARTHRITIS: JOINT PAIN AND ROLE OF IMAGING IN OTHER DISEASE ENTITIES

Although there is abundant literature on structural disease manifestations in OA and associations with pain, far less data are available in regard to structural correlates and pain for other disease entities. Multiple studies have shown that MRI is more sensitive than clinical examination and conventional radiography for the detection of inflammation (i.e., synovitis, bone marrow edema/osteitis, and tenosynovitis) and structural joint damage (i.e., bone erosions and cartilage loss) in patients with rheumatoid arthritis (RA). In routine clinical care, MRI can contribute to an earlier diagnosis of RA, can reveal subclinical disease activity, and can provide information of prognostic significance for the subsequent disease course, which may be useful when deciding the individualized treatment strategy. Commonly, improvement of imaging findings is associated with concomitant improvement in pain. Similarly, in axial or peripheral spondyloarthropathies or other rheumatic conditions, MRI may be very helpful to confirm the diagnosis in an early disease stage as it enables visualization of potential painful structural changes such as enthesitis, osteitis, and synovitis and to initiate consequent targeted treatment.

As joint pain may be nonspecific and often difficult to localize clinically, MRI is able to elucidate potential pain triggers, which may be particularly helpful in hip- or groin-related disorders as these comprise a multitude of possible structural correlates.

Further, imaging has become part of several diagnostic disease definitions in rheumatology. However, it needs to be emphasized that for all disease entities, the challenge remains to establish direct correlations between symptoms and structural damage due to the common nonspecificity and the individual differences of pain perception.

## CONCLUSIONS

OA is assessed radiographically either by semiquantitative scoring systems such as the KL grading scale or by the OARSI atlas, which grades tibiofemoral JSN and osteophytes separately for each compartment. In addition, quantitative JSW measurements can be accomplished either manually or in (semi-) automated fashion.

MRI may be evaluated by semiquantitative scoring approaches, by 3D segmentation, or using compositional techniques. Several MRI scoring systems are available for the assessment of OA, with each having advantages and disadvantages. For assessment of synovitis, CE MRI enables more accurate evaluation than scoring of nonenhanced MRI data. Cartilage or meniscus quantification requires segmentation and exploits the three-dimensional nature of MRI data sets to evaluate tissue dimensions (such as thickness, areas volume, and others) as continuous variables. Compositional MRI techniques allow visualization of the biochemical properties of different joint tissues. It is, therefore, very sensitive to early, premorphologic changes that cannot be seen on conventional MRI. Its role for elucidating associations with pain incidence, progression, or fluctuation needs to be shown.

In population-based studies, a significant discordance between radiographically diagnosed OA and knee pain has been reported. While radiographic evidence of joint damage predisposes to joint pain, the underlying pathologies leading to pain cannot be readily discerned from radiography alone and may require consideration of other factors. Novel study designs are one approach to deal with the so-called structure–symptom discordance. Utilizing imaging modalities such as MRI, several structural alterations such as meniscal tears, subchondral BMLs, subarticular bone attrition, synovitis, and effusion have been related to knee pain. Furthermore, changes in BMLs and inflammatory markers on MRI are associated with fluctuations in pain in patients with knee OA. How much of the variance in pain is accounted for by structural change is not fully understood. One reason for this difficulty is that most studies focused on late disease stages when numerous pathologic changes are already commonly present. In fact, abnormalities on MRI are very common even in knees that are considered to be radiographically normal.

Evidence suggests that large BMLs are strongly associated with knee pain, followed by synovitis and effusion, and potentially also cartilage volume and thickness. Interpretation of these relationships is challenging as it is not clear as to whether all of these associations are truly causal, or rather are markers of the severity of other structural pathology that may be contributing to the pain experience.

## REFERENCES

1. Altman RD, Gold GE. Atlas of individual radiographic features in osteoarthritis, revised. Osteoarthritis Cartilage 2007;15:A1–56.
2. Baker K, Grainger A, Niu J, Clancy M, Guermazi A, Crema M, Hughes L, Buckwalter J, Wooley A, Nevitt M, Felson DT. Relation of synovitis to knee pain using contrast-enhanced MRIs. Ann Rheum Dis 2010;69:1779–83.
3. Cotofana S, Wyman BT, Benichou O, Dreher D, Nevitt M, Gardiner J, Wirth W, Hitzl W, Kwoh CK, Eckstein F, Frobell RB. Relationship between knee pain and the presence, location, size and phenotype of femorotibial denuded areas of subchondral bone as visualized by MRI. Osteoarthritis Cartilage 2013;21:1214–22.
4. Dunlop DD, Manheim LM, Song J, Chang RW. Arthritis prevalence and activity limitations in older adults. Arthritis Rheum 2001;44:212–21.
5. Dye SF, Vaupel GL, Dye CC. Conscious neurosensory mapping of the internal structures of the human knee without intraarticular anesthesia. Am J Sports Med 1998;26:773–7.
6. Englund M, Niu J, Guermazi A, Roemer FW, Hunter DJ, Lynch JA, Lewis CE, Torner J, Nevitt MC, Zhang YQ, Felson DT. Effect of meniscal damage on the development of frequent knee pain, aching, or stiffness. Arthritis Rheum 2007;56:4048–54.
7. Felson DT, Chaisson CE, Hill CL, Totterman SM, Gale ME, Skinner KM, Kazis L, Gale DR. The association of bone marrow lesions with pain in knee osteoarthritis. Ann Intern Med 2001;134:541–9.
8. Felson DT, Niu J, Guermazi A, Roemer F, Aliabadi P, Clancy M, Torner J, Lewis CE, Nevitt MC. Correlation of the development of knee pain with enlarging bone marrow lesions on magnetic resonance imaging. Arthritis Rheum 2007;56:2986–92.

9. Felson DT, Niu J, Guermazi A, Sack B, Aliabadi P. Defining radiographic incidence and progression of knee osteoarthritis: suggested modifications of the Kellgren and Lawrence scale. Ann Rheum Dis 2011;70:1884–6.
10. Guermazi A, Roemer FW, Haugen IK, Crema MD, Hayashi D. MRI-based semi-quantitative scoring of joint pathology in osteoarthritis. Nat Rev Rheumatol 2013;9:236–51.
11. Hannan MT, Felson DT, Pincus T. Analysis of the discordance between radiographic changes and knee pain in osteoarthritis of the knee. J Rheumatol 2000;27:1513–7.
12. Hill CL, Gale DG, Chaisson CE, Skinner K, Kazis L, Gale ME, Felson DT. Knee effusions, popliteal cysts, and synovial thickening: association with knee pain in osteoarthritis. J Rheumatol 2001;28:1330–7.
13. Hunter DJ, Guermazi A, Lo GH, Grainger AJ, Conaghan PG, Boudreau RM, Roemer FW. Evolution of semi-quantitative whole joint assessment of knee OA: MOAKS (MRI Osteoarthritis Knee Score). Osteoarthritis Cartilage 2011;19:990–1002.
14. Hunter DJ, Zhang W, Conaghan PG, Hirko K, Menashe L, Li L, Reichmann WM, Losina E. Systematic review of the concurrent and predictive validity of MRI biomarkers in OA. Osteoarthritis Cartilage 2011;19:557–88.
15. Kellgren JH, Lawrence JS. Radiological assessment of osteo-arthrosis. Ann Rheum Dis 1957;16:494–502.
16. Kornaat PR, Bloem JL, Ceulemans RY, Riyazi N, Rosendaal FR, Nelissen RG, Carter WO, Hellio Le Graverand MP, Kloppenburg M. Osteoarthritis of the knee: association between clinical features and MR imaging findings. Radiology 2006;239:811–7.
17. Neogi T, Felson D, Niu J, Nevitt M, Lewis CE, Aliabadi P, Sack B, Torner J, Bradley L, Zhang Y. Association between radiographic features of knee osteoarthritis and pain: results from two cohort studies. BMJ 2009;339:b2844.
18. Roemer FW, Hayes CW, Miller CG, Hoover K, Guermazi A. Imaging atlas for eligibility and on-study safety of potential knee adverse events in anti-NGF studies (Part 1). Osteoarthritis Cartilage 2015;23:S22–42.
19. Roemer FW, Nevitt MC, Felson DT, Niu J, Lynch JA, Crema MD, Lewis CE, Torner J, Guermazi A. Predictive validity of within-grade scoring of longitudinal changes of MRI-based cartilage morphology and bone marrow lesion assessment in the tibio-femoral joint—the MOST study. Osteoarthritis Cartilage 2012;20:1391–8.
20. Zhang Y, Nevitt M, Niu J, Lewis C, Torner J, Guermazi A, Roemer F, McCulloch C, Felson DT. Fluctuation of knee pain and changes in bone marrow lesions, effusions, and synovitis on magnetic resonance imaging. Arthritis Rheum 2011;63:691–9.

CHAPTER 7

# Assessing Joint Pain and Function in the Clinic

*Lisa C. Carlesso, Gillian A. Hawker, Jacqueline R. Hochman, and Aileen M. Davis*

The purpose of this chapter is to provide an overview of available generic and disease-specific measures of joint pain and function that can be easily used in the clinical setting. It is often difficult to disentangle the concept of function from pain when measured in joints, and there are several clinical observational and physical tests that can help clarify the relationship between the two. This chapter focuses solely on the use of patient-reported questionnaires that pertain to the peripheral joints. Measures of pain will be presented first that address pain intensity and pain quality, including neuropathic components. Measures of function will be presented next, focusing on generic and disease- and joint-specific questionnaires. Keeping in mind the need for efficiency in a clinical setting, we have chosen to present, where available and appropriate, the shortened version of measures. For each measure, the content, application, and relevant measurement properties are presented to help facilitate the choice of the most appropriate measure for one's clinical practice. Psychometrics for all measures are presented in Tables 7-1 and 7-2. The reliability, validity, and ability to detect change are summarized. Where available, evidence for various patient conditions/groups is also provided. In clinical practice, as measurement is focused on the individual, it is critical that measures

TABLE 7-1 **Psychometric Properties: Pain Measures**

| Measure | Reliability | Validity | Detection of Change and Interpretability |
|---|---|---|---|
| Visual analog scale | Test–retest ICC:<br>Literate and illiterate rheumatology outpatients: $r = 0.94$ and 0.71, respectively) [36]<br>Patients with acute pain: $r = 0.97$ [19] | Construct validity:<br>Scores correlated with other pain measures $r = 0.62–0.91$ [30]<br>>30 mm = moderate pain rating<br>>54 mm = severe pain rating [26] | MCID:<br>Rotator cuff disease 1.4 cm on 10 cm pain VAS [76]<br>Hip and knee OA: 15.3–19.9 mm on 100 mm VAS [77] |
| Numeric rating scale | Test–retest ICC:<br>Literate and illiterate rheumatology outpatients: $r = 0.96$ and 0.95, respectively [36]<br>Patients with shoulder pain: $r = 0.74$ [60] | Construct validity:<br>Correlated to VAS in patients with rheumatic and other chronic pain conditions ($r > 0.86$) [36] | A reduction of 2 points, or 30% is clinically important in chronic LBP, OA, postherpetic neuralgia [35]<br>Shoulder pain MCID 2.17 [59] |
| Short-Form McGill Pain Questionnaire | Internal consistency:<br>Cronbach's α in rheumatology population: 0.73–0.89 [23]<br>Test–retest ICC: −0.45 to 0.73 at 1 and 3 months; 1–3 days: 0.79–0.93 [74]<br>= 0.89 SF-MPQ, VAS average pain and total scores [43] | Content validity:<br>Mean intensity scores ranged from 1.57 to 2.60 in rheumatology patients [23]<br>Hip and knee OA patients, correlated with WOMAC and SF-36 bodily pain scales: $r = 0.36$ and >0.36, respectively [40] | MSK patients: SRM = 0.80 [74]<br>OA population: MDC for total, sensory, affective, average, and current pain = 5.2, 4.5, 2.8, 1.4, 1.4 cm, respectively [43] |
| ICOAP | Internal $\alpha$<br>Cronbach's α = 0.93 in hip and knee OA subjects [45] | Construct validity: $r = 0.60$ for KOOS 0.81–0.91 for WOMAC [45, 52] | Knee OA: SRMs 0.49–0.58 [21, 65] 1.67 [42] |

| | | | |
|---|---|---|---|
| | Test–retest ICC in hip and knee OA subjects: 0.57–0.85 [45, 52, 65, 71] | Predictive validity: over 2 years, constant ($B$ = 0.484; $P$ = 0.001) and intermittent ($B$ = 0.104; $P$ = 0.040) pain = to decreased WOMAC-PF. Increased constant pain ($B$ = 0.077; $P$ = 0.001) = to decreased chair stand test performance in women. High baseline intermittent pain = to poor performance on repeated chair stands ($B$ = 0.035; $P$ = 0.021), baseline constant pain = to poor 400-m walk performance in women ($B$ = 0.636; $P$ = 0.047) [29] | Hip OA: SRMs 0.11– 0.19 [21]<br>Knee replacement: SRMs 0.84–1.02<br>Hip replacement: SRMs 1.50–2.29 [27]<br>MCID knee OA 18.5 [71] |
| PainDETECT | Internal consistency:<br>Cronbach's $\alpha$ = average 0.76 across 6 conditions with NP: spinal cord injury 0.63, chronic low back pain 0.76, human immunodeficiency virus-related 0.82, small fiber neuropathy 0.74, diabetic peripheral neuropathy 0.78, posttrauma/postsurgical 0.78 [25] | Discriminant validity of 6 pain conditions with all pain symptom items (0.3–0.7), but two nonsensory items (<0.3)<br>Mean scores of 15.2, 19.8, and 24.0 = mild, moderate, and severe pain cut scores of the BPI-SF, respectively [24]<br>Sensitivity, 64%; specificity, 62% in people with neck/upper limb pain [75]<br>Sensitivity, 85%; specificity, 83% in people with CLBP [39]<br>Knee OA-higher scores associated with lower PPT scores $\rho$ = −0.32 to −0.35 and S-LANSS $r$ = 0.64; agreement with S-LANSS on cut scores for classification of NP $\kappa$ = 0.33–0.46 [61] | ES for mild, moderate, and severe pain:<br>Mild vs. moderate −0.56<br>Mild vs. severe −1.13<br>Moderate vs. severe −0.57<br>Negative values = less neuropathic pain in the group with the lower level of average pain severity [24] |
| S-LANSS | Internal consistency:<br>Cronbach's $\alpha$ = 0.76 and 0.80 [18] | Sensitivity, 73–79% and specificity, 75–80% with pain types identified by clinical examination.<br>Discriminant validity: Presence of NP—clinician rating and S-LANSS score: $r$ = 0.54<br>Convergent validity: NP scale and PainDETECT [18]<br>Knee OA: poor correlation with PPT testing [61] | No known data; however, main purpose is to screen for NP |

*Abbreviations*: ICC, intraclass correlation; VAS, visual analog scale; MCID, minimum clinically important difference; NRS, numeric rating scale; OA, osteoarthritis; WOMAC, Western Ontario and McMaster Universities Osteoarthritis Index; ES, effect size; SF-MPQ, Short-Form MPQ; ICC, intraclass correlation coefficient; MSK, musculoskeletal; SRM, standardized response mean; NSF, Norwegian Short Form; 95% CI, 95% confidence interval; SF-36 BPS, Short-Form 36 Bodily Pain Scale; RA, rheumatoid arthritis; OA, osteoarthritis; MDC, minimal detectable change; ICOAP, Measure of Intermittent and Constant Osteoarthritis Pain; KOOS, Knee Injury and Osteoarthritis Outcome Score; SRM, standardized response mean; BPI-SF, Brief Pain Inventory short form; NP, neuropathic pain; PPT, pressure pain threshold; CLBP, chronic low back pain; S-LANSS, Self-Reported Version of the Leeds Assessment of Neuropathic Signs and Symptoms.

TABLE 7-2 **Psychometric Properties: Function Measures**

| Measure | Reliability | Validity | Detection of Change and Interpretability |
|---|---|---|---|
| HAQ-II | Internal consistency in RA patients: Cronbach's $\alpha = 0.88$ [81] | Concurrent validity: original HAQ ($r = 0.92$), SF-36 PFS ($r = -0.85$), EuroQol ($r = -0.67$), Rheumatology Distress Index ($r = 0.61$), Rheumatoid Arthritis Disease Activity Index ($r = 0.65$), and Arthritis Impact Measurement Scales depression and anxiety scales ($r = 0.44$ and 0.38, respectively) [81]<br>Predictive validity: correlated with clinical outcomes of pain, fatigue, patient's and physician's assessments of global disease severity, Disease Activity Score in 28 joints, erythrocyte sedimentation rate, joint counts, medical costs, joint replacement, and work disability [81] | Has substantially less floor effects than original HAQ; no data on responsiveness [81] |
| SPADI | Internal consistency: Cronbach's $\alpha = 0.86$–0.98 [3, 64]<br>Test–retest ICC = 0.86–0.95 [9, 69] | Construct validity with other measures:<br>DASH $r = 0.55$–0.93 [10, 73]<br>SF-36 PCS: 0.63 and 0.67 [10, 12]<br>Active ROM: 0.54–0.80 and 0.38 [64, 78]<br>SF-36 mental: 0.08 [10]<br>NPRS: $r = 0.49$–0.67 [63] | MCID: 8–23.1 points [32, 68, 69]<br>ES and SRMs of total score:<br>Total shoulder arthroplasty: ES 2.10, SRM 1.72 [7]<br>Adhesive capsulitis: steroids: ES 1.20–1.94, SRM 1.27–1.81 [78]<br>Shoulder pain, physiotherapy: ES 1.26, SRM 1.38 [47]<br>Rotator cuff surgery: SRM 1.23 [12]<br>Various upper extremity, occupational, physiotherapy: ES 0.80, SRM 0.67 [69]<br>General practice, conservative therapy: ES 0.34 [80] |

| | | | |
|---|---|---|---|
| QuickDASH | Internal consistency: Cronbach's $\alpha = 0.90–0.94$ [14]<br>Test–retest ICC = 0.91–0.94 [14, 60] | Convergent validity with VAS of overall problem $r = 0.70$; overall pain $r = 0.73$; ability to function $r = 0.80$; ability to work $r = 0.76$ [13, 14, 67]<br>Known groups mean scores: able to do all needed to vs. limited = 25.4 vs. 48.6; able to work vs. unable to work due to upper limb problem mean scores = 27.5 vs. 52.6 [14] | MCID = 8.0–15.91 [38, 60]<br>Total shoulder arthroplasty: ES 1.26 [8]<br>Shoulder or hand: conservative treatment: SRM 0.79 [14]<br>Various upper extremity surgery: SRM 0.63–1.1 [44, 54] |
| WOMAC | Knee OA: Internal consistency: Cronbach's $\alpha$.<br>Pain: 0.62–0.96<br>Stiffness: 0.65–0.94<br>Function: 0.61–0.98 [53, 79]<br>Test–retest ICC:<br>Pain: 0.62–0.98<br>Stiffness: 0.52–0.89<br>Function: 0.61–0.97 [82] | Convergent validity—moderate to strong correlations with similar measures hip and knee OA and hip and knee arthroplasty (e.g., NRS, SF-36 physical subscales) [34, 41, 62, 72, 82] | Large effects for up to 2 years post-TJR<br>Post-TKR: 1.7 function 1.2 pain [27, 28]<br>Post-THR: 1.7 function 2.6 pain [27, 28] |
| | Hip OA: Internal consistency: Cronbach's $\alpha$.<br>Pain: 0.81–0.90<br>Stiffness: 0.77–0.86<br>Function: 0.94–0.96 [11, 53] | Moderate to strong correlations with performance measures for hip and knee OA and hip and knee arthroplasty (e.g., walking, stair climbing, rising from a chair) [2, 20, 37, 41] | MCID for TKR (up to 2 years postoperatively; for pain 22.9–36, for stiffness 14.4–21.4, for function 19–33 [33] |
| | Test–retest ICC:<br>Pain: 0.81–0.90<br>Stiffness: 0.77–0.86<br>Function: 0.93–0.94 [11, 53] | Divergent validity: low correlations with dissimilar measures (e.g., SF-36 mental subscales) [82] | CID for THR 1 year: 41 pain, 34 function (out of 100)<br>Treatment with NSAIDs:<br>SRMs for function: hip OA 0.49; knee OA 0.64 [62]<br>MCII for function: hip OA 33.4; knee OA 28.4 [62] |

(*continued*)

TABLE 7-2 **Psychometric Properties: Function Measures (*continued*)**

| Measure | Reliability | Validity | Detection of Change and Interpretability |
|---|---|---|---|
| AUSCAN | Internal consistency: Cronbach's $\alpha = 0.90–0.98$<br>0.90–0.94 for Likert scale<br>0.94–0.98 for VAS<br>Test–retest ICCs: 0.70–86 for Likert scale and 0.94–0.98 for the VAS [17] | Construct validity OA population correlation with measures of grip, pinch, pain, global function, physician-rated severity, the FIHOA, the HAQ for the Likert scale ranged from 0.33 to 0.82 and for the VAS ranged from 0.51 to 0.86 [17] | SRMs of AUSCAN with FIHOA −0.74 to −0.23 for Likert scale and −0.84 to −0.39 for VAS [17]<br>Every 1-unit increase in AUSCAN functional scale is equal to decrease in grip or pinch strength, 0.19 and 1.13 kg, respectively, and, therefore, can correspond to changes in strength [1] |
| AAOS-FAM | Internal consistency: Cronbach's $\alpha$ total scale = 0.93; subscales 0.91, 0.83, 0.61, and 0.88 for pain, function, stiffness, and giving way subscales, respectively.<br>Test–retest = 0.79 for total scale; subscales 0.87, 0.81, 0.99, and 0.81 for pain, function, stiffness, and giving way subscales, respectively. | Discriminant validity correlated with physician assessments and questionnaire for pain ($r = 0.49$) and function ($r = 0.43$). Patient responses strongly correlated with SF-36 scores ($r = 0.65$) and assessment of the lower extremity core ($r = 0.89$) [4] | No data reported for the global foot and ankle module; however, overall lower extremity scores correlate ($r = 0.54$) with changes in physician-assessed function scores, indicating responsiveness to change [4] |

*Abbreviations*: VAS, visual analog scale; MCID, minimum clinically important difference; NRS, numeric rating scale; OA, osteoarthritis; HAQ-II, Health Assessment Questionnaire II; AUSCAN, Australia Canadian Hand Osteoarthritis Index; AAOS-FAM, American Academy of Orthopedic Surgeons Lower Limb Outcomes Assessment: Foot and Ankle Module; WOMAC, Western Ontario and McMaster Universities Osteoarthritis Index; DASH, Disabilities of the Arm, Shoulder, and Hand; NSAIDs, nonsteroidal anti-inflammatory drugs; ES, effect size; TKR, total knee replacement; ICC, intraclass correlation coefficient; MSK, musculoskeletal; SRM, standardized response mean; NSF, Norwegian Short Form; 95% CI, 95% confidence interval; RA, rheumatoid arthritis; MDC, minimal detectable change; OA, osteoarthritis; FIHOA, Functional Index of Hand OA; MCII, minimal clinically important improvement.

have clinical utility, validity representing the aspect of pain or function for which it is intended, and high reliability to limit measurement error such that clinical change can be detected.

# PAIN MEASURES

## Intensity

### Visual Analog Scale

A unidimensional measure of pain, the visual analog scale (VAS), has been used to measure pain in a number of populations [57]. It is a continuous single-item scale that employs a horizontal or a vertical line, typically 100 mm in length with anchors at either end with two verbal descriptors representing each extreme of the symptom [50]. Intermediate anchors and descriptors are not recommended to avoid clustering of scores around a preferred number. The descriptors are typically *no pain* (score of 0) and *worst imaginable pain* or *pain as bad as it can be* (score of 100) [50]. Recall period varies but is most commonly reported to capture current pain or pain within the past 24 hours.

The VAS is freely available in the public domain and can be found by conducting an online search. Graphical formats can be obtained from Scott and Huskisson [70]. Patients are asked to place a line perpendicular to the VAS at the point that best represents their pain intensity. The score is then determined by using a ruler and measuring the distance from the *no pain* anchor to the patients' mark [50]. A higher score indicates a higher intensity of pain. The following cut points were established with postsurgical patients following a variety of procedures: no pain, 0–4 mm; mild pain, 5–44 mm; moderate pain, 45–74 mm; and severe pain, 75–100 mm [49]. For patients with chronic musculoskeletal (MSK) pain, VAS scores on a 10mm scale of $<3.4$ were described for mild pain, 3.5 to 7.4 for moderate pain, and $>7.5$ for severe pain [22]. Respondent burden is minimal as it takes $<1$ minute to complete; however, administration is limited to paper and pencil methods, thereby not allowing verbal or phone or electronic administration. Also, it has been noted that the length of the scale can change when photocopying;

so caution should be exercised when doing so [50]. The format can also affect the score, as slightly lower scores have been reported with use of a horizontal line compared with a vertical. For this reason, the same format should be used within each patient. The number of translations has been numerous for cross-cultural adaptation. Psychometrics for all pain measures are presented in Table 7-1.

### Numeric Rating Scale

The numeric rating scale (NRS) is another unidimensional single-item measure of pain intensity used in adult populations [66]. The most commonly used version consists of an 11-point scale in which patients select a rating between 0 and 10 to indicate their pain intensity. It is often presented as a horizontal line or bar with similar anchors to the VAS, referring to extreme states of pain [66]. For the NRS, 0 typically represents *no pain*, while 10 represents the *worst imaginable pain* or *pain as bad as it can be*. The recall period varies, but often patients are asked to report average pain intensity or pain in the last 24 hours [31].

The NRS is freely available and can be found by conducting an online search or at http://partnersagainstpain.com/measuring-pain/assessment-tool/#pain_intensity. Its administration can be done graphically or verbally, thereby allowing use on the telephone [50]. The patient is asked to indicate the numeric value between 0 and 10 that best represents their pain intensity, with higher scores representing higher pain intensity. The number indicated by the patients that corresponds to their pain is recorded. Respondent burden is minimal at <1 minute. Because of ease of use and minimal translation difficulties, cross-cultural adaptation has occurred widely. See Table 7-1 for psychometric information.

## Quality: Sensory and Affective

### Short-Form McGill Pain Questionnaire

The Short-Form McGill Pain Questionnaire (SF-MPQ) is a shortened version of the MPQ. It is a multidimensional questionnaire designed to measure sensory and affective aspects of pain as well as pain intensity in adults with chronic pain [58]. Two subscales comprise the Pain Rating Index, represented by 11 words on the sensory subscale and 4 words on the affective subscale [58]. The questionnaire also includes one item for Present Pain intensity, and an item is scored on a 10-cm VAS for average pain [58]. Recall period is the present time. The questionnaire is commonly used to discriminate among different types of syndromes [58].

The SF-MPQ is freely available from the developer, Ronald Melzack, and online at http://www.physio-pedia.com/Short-form_McGill_Pain_Questionnaire. A search on the internet identified that the questionnaire is posted by several clinical sites. For each of the words in the Pain Rating Index, the patient identifies a score between 0 (none) and 3 (severe) [58]. The total for the Pain Rating Index is the sum of all scores, with a possible range of 0–45. The Present Pain scale and the VAS scores range from 0 to 5 and 0 to 10. Higher scores indicate worse pain. No established cut points exist. The burden is minimal at 2–5 minutes for completion and approximately 1 minute to score. The SF-MPQ has been translated into the following languages: English, French, Amharic, Chinese, Czech, Danish, Farsi, Greek, Hebrew, Hindi, Korean, Norwegian, Swedish, Thai, and Turkish [46]. See Table 7-1 for psychometric information.

## Quality: Intermittent and Constant Pain

### Intermittent and Constant Osteoarthritis Pain

The Intermittent and Constant Osteoarthritis Pain (ICOAP) was designed as a multidimensional measure to evaluate the pain experience of people with hip and knee osteoarthritis (OA). A version is available for each population. The scale includes items that pertain to pain intensity and frequency, as well as its impact on mood, sleep, and quality of life, all independent of pain-related function [45]. It is an 11-item scale that evaluates two domains, constant and intermittent pain [45]. In addition, there are two supplementary items that evaluate the predictability of intermittent pain [21]. All items are constructed on a 5-point rating scale, with responses ranging from *not at all* to *extremely* in regards to pain intensity and from *never* to *very often* for pain frequency [45]. The responses for the two supplementary items range from *never* to *very often*. The recall period is one week [21].

The ICOAP and user guide can be obtained freely on the Osteoarthritis Research Society International website www.oarsi.org. The measure is interviewer administered either in person or by telephone [45]. Items are scored from 0 to 4, and totals for subscales are produced separately. Rules for how to deal with missing items are also provided. The scores are then normalized from 0 (no pain) to 100 (extreme pain). No scoring guidelines for the two supplementary items are available. Higher scores indicate a worse pain experience. The measure takes <10 minutes to complete and is easy to administer. To date, the scale has been translated into multiple languages, and all translated versions are available at www.oarsi.org. See Table 7-1 for psychometric information.

## Neuropathic Pain

### PainDETECT

The PainDETECT questionnaire is a measure that was originally developed to distinguish neuropathic from non-neuropathic pain among people with low back pain [39]. It has also been used to identify a neuropathic component to peripheral joint pain [61]. The questionnaire consists of nine questions. The first seven questions are about the presence and severity of neuropathic pain qualities. The eighth question assesses the pattern of pain. The ninth question asks about the presence or absence of radiating pain [39]. Since its development, four additional questions have been added to address pain severity, currently and in the past 4 weeks, and the presence of radiating pain by marking pain distribution on a body manikin [56]. These questions do not factor into the scoring. The recall period is the current time period or the last 4 weeks [39].

The PainDETECT is available as part of the original article. It is patient administered by paper and pencil and can be easily completed in 5 minutes. The first seven questions (pain quality) are scored from 0 (never) to 5 (very strongly). The pain pattern is scored from −1 to 2 depending on which pattern is chosen, and radiating pain is scored as either 2 (yes) or 0 (no). The total score can range from −1 to 38 and is interpreted in terms of the likelihood of neuropathic pain. Scores <12 indicate that a neuropathic component to the pain is less likely (>15%), whereas scores >19 suggest that the presence of neuropathic pain is highly likely (>90%) [39]. Scores in between these values suggest uncertainty, but there may be a neuropathic component to the pain. A search on PubMed identified that the scale has been translated into several languages, including Japanese, Turkish, Dutch, and Spanish. See Table 7-1 for psychometric information.

## Self-Reported Version of the Leeds Assessment of Neuropathic Signs and Symptoms

The Self-Reported Version of the Leeds Assessment of Neuropathic Signs and Symptoms (S-LANSS) is a modified version (to facilitate self-report) of the original LANSS pain scale [18]. It is designed to identify people with neuropathic pain and, thus, uses a cut score. Seven items from the original scale are available, besides additional modifications of a body map for identifying pain sites areas and an 11-point NRS asking patients to rate "how bad their pain has been in the last week [18]." Items inquire about sensations associated with neuropathic pain such as pins and needles, electric shocks, and burning. Five of the seven items are answered either Yes or No. For the remaining two, patients choose between two options. Answers to different questions have different values. The recall period is one week [18].

The scale is available as part of the original article. The scale can be completed in both paper and pencil format or through clinician interview. Scoring for the seven items is weighted with values of 1 (1 item), 2 (1 item), 3 (2 items), or 5 (3 items). The NRS item scale is anchored from 0 (no pain) to 10 (pain as severe as it could be). To obtain a score, each of the seven items is summed. The body map and the NRS rating are not included in the scoring. A score of >12 indicates the pain of predominantly neuropathic origin [18]. The scale is easy to use and can be completed in ~5 minutes. A search on PubMed identified that the scale has been translated into Greek, Swedish, Turkish, Arabic, Chinese, and Korean. See Table 7-1 for psychometric information.

# FUNCTION MEASURES

## General and Inflammatory Arthritis

### Health Assessment Questionnaire II (HAQ-II)

A modified version of the original Health Assessment Questionnaire (HAQ) that was developed to assess functional status in adults with arthritis, this unidimensional scale was designed to improve clinical use [81]. Items are scored on a 4-point Likert scale ranging from 0 (without difficulty) to 3 (unable to do). Ten items referring to various activities, including rising from a chair, walking, toileting, reaching, waiting in line, opening doors, stairs, outdoor chores, lifting, and moving heavy objects, are available. Five of the items are from the original HAQ, and five are new [81]. The recall period is 1 week.

The questionnaire is most commonly self-administered, but can be interviewer administered. It is freely available from the developer online at https://www.arthritis-research.org/sites/default/files/HAQII.pdf. It is quick and easy to use and can be completed in ~5 minutes. The score is obtained by summing the scored items, a minimum of 8 out of 10, and dividing them by the number completed. The score ranges from 0 to 3.0, with higher scores indicating worse function. The scores are nonlinear, meaning that a change in score from 1 to 2 is not the same amount as a change from 2 to 3 [6]. The HAQ-II is also available in Dutch [55]. See Table 7-2 for psychometric information.

# ASSESSMENT BY BODY AREA

## Shoulder

### Shoulder Pain and Disability Index

The Shoulder Pain and Disability Index (SPADI) was developed for use in an outpatient setting to measure the impact of shoulder pathology in terms of pain and disability [64]. It has 13 items, 5 pertaining to pain and 8 for function. All items are originally scored on a VAS, ranging from no pain/no difficulty to worst pain imaginable/so difficult required help [64]. An NRS version was created later to improve ease of use, with ratings for each item ranging from 0 (best) to 10 (worst) [9]. The recall period is 1 week.

Free online at https://www.tac.vic.gov.au/files-to-move/media/upload/spi.pdf; it is easy and short to complete in ~2 to 3 minutes. Scoring was originally performed by summing the items. At least, 11 of 13 items must be completed for the total score. The total score is the mean of the pain and function subscores [64]. Later, the *2/3 missing rule* was applied, requiring at least 3 of 5 pain and 6 of 8 function items completed for each of the subscales to be valid [9]. Higher scores indicate worse pain and function. The SPADI has been translated into several languages, including Norwegian, German, Slovene, Chinese, Hindi, Brazilian Portuguese, Japanese, Turkish, and French Canadian [55]. See Table 7-2 for psychometric information.

## Disabilities of the Arm, Shoulder, and Hand (DASH) (Shortened Version QuickDASH)

The QuickDASH is a self-reported measure for disorders of the upper extremity. The measure is region specific, not joint specific. The QuickDASH has 11 items (3 for symptoms, 8 for function) as well as two optional modules consisting of 4 items to measure high performance sport/music or work [14]. The optional modules are intended for athletes, performing artists, and workers whose jobs require high levels of physical performance. All items are scored on a Likert scale [14]. Recall period for the items is 1 week.

The measure is the property and copyright of the Institute for Work and Health, and it is freely available at (http://www.dash.iwh.on.ca/). Scoring is relatively easy. The items are scored ranging from 1 (no difficulty/symptoms) to 5 (extreme difficulty [unable to do]/symptoms). For the disability/symptom subscale, at least 10 of the 11 items are necessary for the total score (3 of 3 for symptoms and 7 of 8 for function) [14]. The values of all completed responses are summed and averaged, with possible scores from 1 to 5. This value is then transformed to a score out of 100 by subtracting one and multiplying by 25. A higher score indicates greater disability. If more than one item is left blank, the disability/symptom score cannot be calculated. The optional modules are scored as above, but all four questions must be answered to calculate the score. Respondent burden is minimal at <5 minutes to complete [14]. All items are easy to understand. The QuickDASH is currently available in 27 approved translations [48]. See Table 7-2 for psychometric information.

## Hip and Knee

### Western Ontario and McMaster Universities Osteoarthritis Index Version 5.0

The Western Ontario and McMaster Universities Osteoarthritis Index (WOMAC) was designed to assess the course of disease in people with hip or knee OA. It is available in multiple formats, including a 5-point Likert scale, 100-mm VAS, and 11-box NRS. It is a multidimensional scale with three subscales: (1) pain with activities, (2) stiffness, and (3) disability [16]. The measure has 24 items, with 5, 2, and 17 items, respectively, per subscale. The Likert-scaled version has five anchors for each question, ranging from 0 (none) to 4 (extreme). The VAS and NRS versions allow for answers to be selected between 0 and 100 mm or 0 and 10 box scales, with the far left of the scale representing *none* and the far right *extreme* [5]. The recall period is 48 hours.

The measure is available from the author, Professor Nicholas Bellamy (e-mail: n.bellamy@uq.edu.au). Information regarding use and permission for clinical use can be found at www.womac.org. The measure is self-administered or can also be completed in an interview format. It has been validated for several modes, including face-to-face, telephone, and electronically [5]. For the Likert version of the scale, the total score ranges from 0 to 96 and is calculated by summing the response to each item in each subscale. The totals for the subscales range from 0 to 20 for pain, 0 to 8 for stiffness, and 0 to 68 for physical activity. For the VAS format, the ranges are 0–500 for pain, 0–200 for stiffness, and 0–1700 for physical function [5]. When two or more items in the pain or stiffness sections or four or more items in the physical activity sections are missed, the subscales should not be summed and are considered invalid and do not contribute to the overall score [15]. Higher scores indicate worse OA-related symptoms of pain, stiffness, and physical function. The scale takes approximately ~10 minutes to complete and is easy to score. Translation has occurred in more than 100 languages [16]. The psychometrics of the WOMAC have been extensively evaluated. Because of the large body of evidence, studies reflecting the general results are provided in Table 7-2.

## Hand

### Australia Canadian Hand Osteoarthritis Index (AUSCAN)

The multidimensional Australia Canadian Hand Osteoarthritis Index (AUSCAN) scale was designed as a self-report measure for the assessment of hand pain, stiffness, and function in persons with OA [17]. Similar to the WOMAC, there are three subscales, including pain (5 items), stiffness (1 item), and function (9 items) for a total of 15 items. Pain is assessed at rest and with activities that include gripping, lifting, turning, and squeezing objects. Stiffness is assessed in reference to the sensation upon waking. The function items ask about difficulty turning, fastening, opening, carrying, grabbing, and squeezing various objects [17]. Three response formats are available, a Likert-scaled version, a VAS format, and a NRS http://auscan.org/auscan/index.htm. The recall period is 48 hours.

The scale is available from Dr. Bellamy (e-mail: n.bellamy@uq.edu.au). It is copyrighted, and its cost is unknown. The scale is administered in either a patient or clinician questionnaire and can also be done via the telephone. The Likert scale responses range from 0 (none) to 4 (extreme), the VAS from 0 to 100 mm, and the NRS from 0 to 10, with higher values indicating more extreme responses. The total score is calculated by summing all items from each of the three subscales. No instructions for handling missing values are available. Higher total scores indicate worse status. Respondent burden is minimal, with a completion time of ~5 minutes. Translations and adaptations have occurred in more than 30 languages http://auscan.org/auscan/index.htm. See Table 7-2 for psychometric information.

## Foot

### American Academy of Orthopedic Surgeons Lower Limb Outcomes Assessment: Foot and Ankle Module (AAOS-FAM)

This multidimensional scale is designed to evaluate the patient's perception of his or her foot and ankle health. It contains 25 questions with two subscales exist: core consisting of pain (nine questions), function (six questions), stiffness and swelling (two questions), giving way (three questions), and the shoe comfort subscale (five questions). Responses for the first four subscales are given on a scale of 1–5, 1–6, or 1–7. The lowest number (1) indicates the best outcome and the highest (5, 6, or 7) the worst. Responses for the shoe comfort subscale are Yes, No, or Not applicable [4]. The recall period for items is 1 week.

The scale including scoring instructions and the spreadsheet to calculate scores is freely available on the AAOS website without copyright or registration at URL: http://www.aaos.org/research/outcomes/outcomes_lower.asp. Scores are standardized to a percentage (0–100) score and then transformed on normative scale. A lower normative score is indicative of worse foot health relative to the population (2). Scores range from 0 to 100 for each subscale and can be placed on a normative scale from −26 to 56 based on the general population [51]. Respondent burden is not provided. However, some training (self-study of document on website) in the scoring of the measure is required (see URL: http://www.aaos.org/research/outcomes/outcomes_lower.asp). See Table 7-2 for psychometric information.

# DISCUSSION

We have reviewed multiple measures of pain and function for the assessment of joint pain in the clinic. Each has its own strengths and weaknesses, and some are better than others at attaining the desired qualities of a clinical measure (i.e., reliability, validity, and the ability to detect change). For pain, both the VAS and the NRS are unidimensional single-item scales that provide an estimate of a patients' pain intensity. They are easy to administer, complete, and score; however, clinicians may prefer the NRS for its slightly simpler scoring. Neither measure provides a comprehensive evaluation of a patients' pain whether acute, chronic, or neuropathic. Evaluation of these multiple dimensions requires a number of valid and reliable questionnaires. The SF-MPQ is a multidimensional generic pain measure that is useful to describe not only the quantity, but also the quality of the patients' pain. It has demonstrated reliability and validity in rheumatological and osteoarthritic populations and detects change in OA and MSK populations in response to rehabilitation. It is an easier and more efficient version of the original long form, and therefore, it is better suited to the clinical setting. However, sufficient experience is required to adequately complete the SF-MPQ; therefore, new users require supervision during completion [43]. The ICOAP, a measure for patients with hip or knee OA, captures the unique nature of constant and intermittent pain in this population as well as the impact of pain on mood, sleep, and quality of life, separate and distinct from the impact of pain on functioning [45]. The ICOAP is intended for use together with a measure of OA disability. It is reliable and valid, and its ability to detect change is better in those who have had a hip or knee replacement than those with hip or knee OA [21, 27]. Literature regarding assessment of neuropathic pain related to joint problems is relatively less. Of the two measures reviewed for neuropathic pain, it is currently unknown which of the PainDETECT or S-LANSS is better overall for use in patients with joint pain in clinical settings. The PainDETECT was created in patients with chronic low back pain, and the sensitivity and specificity suggest that it is not recommended for use in people with neck or upper limb pain [75]. Compared with the S-LANSS, however, it appears superior for knee OA populations as it was better correlated with pressure pain threshold values [61]. The S-LANSS does not appear to have any data for detecting change, whereas the PainDETECT has effect sizes for mild, moderate, and severe pain [24]. None of the pain measures reviewed is optimal for use in isolation as each covers unique aspects of pain. Further, variability in method of administration, burden, and evidence to support the psychometric properties of each measure suggest that no one pain measure can be recommended for use in all situations. Rather, the aspects of pain that are of interest to measure for each patient should guide the clinician.

The functional measures reviewed include the generic HAQ-II designed for use in rheumatological and osteoarthritic populations. Having minimized the floor effects of the original HAQ [81], it is valid and easy to use clinically, particularly for rheumatological patients. For the upper extremity, The QuickDASH is a general measure for the upper limb and, therefore, cannot provide data for specific joints. That being said, its psychometrics have been assessed across a number of conditions and joint diseases. Its ease of use, minimal burden, and accessibility make it highly recommended. The SPADI is shoulder specific, and like the QuickDASH, it has been tested in multiple conditions and is short, easy to score, and freely available. Although highly responsive (see Table 7-2), it may be limited in the measurement of overhead work or heavy use of the shoulder as there is only one item to assess this type of function. The WOMAC is one of the most commonly used measures for hip and knee dysfunction. While easy to use and score with separate subscale totals, the need to obtain permission for use and pay licensing fees is a barrier to clinic use. Items for the function subscale do not include more physically demanding tasks that may limit measurement of more physically active patients. Of the available foot and ankle measures, the AAOS-FAM is reliable, but is in need of further validation, and importantly, it is lacking data on its ability to detect change. The AUSCAN has been assessed mainly in people with rheumatoid arthritis or OA and is associated with performance measures. Like the WOMAC, it is easy to use and has low burden; however, it is copyrighted, making access difficult. A number of measures of function for joints of the upper and lower extremity have been presented because of their ease of use clinically. They range in their ability to measure general, specific, and multiple joints. Clinicians should consider which approach is preferred for each patient in combination with the measurement properties reviewed to optimize accurate assessment of joint function.

## REFERENCES

1. Allen KD, Jordan JM, Renner JB, Kraus VB. Validity, factor structure, and clinical relevance of the AUSCAN Osteoarthritis Hand Index. Arthritis Rheum 2006;54:551–6.
2. Allyson J, Voaklander D, Johnston D, Suarez-Almazor M. The effect of age on pain, function, and quality of life after total hip and knee arthroplasty. Arch Intern Med 2001;161:454–60.
3. Alsanawi HA, Alghadir A, Anwer S, Roach KE, Alawaji A. Cross-cultural adaptation and psychometric properties of an Arabic version of the Shoulder Pain and Disability Index. Int J Rehabil Res 2015;38:270–75.
4. American Academy of Orthopaedic Surgeons. Foot and ankle module, Vol. 2015. Rosemont, IL: American Academy of Orthopaedic Surgeons; 2015.
5. American College of Rheumatology. Western Ontario and McMaster Universities Osteoarthritis Index, Vol. 2015. Atlanta, GA: American College of Rheumatology; 2015.
6. Anderson J, Sayles H, Curtis JR, Wolfe F, Michaud K. Converting modified health assessment questionnaire (HAQ), multidimensional HAQ, and HAQII scores into original HAQ scores using models developed with a large cohort of rheumatoid arthritis patients. Arthritis Care Res (Hoboken) 2010;62:1481–88.
7. Angst F, Goldhahn J, Drerup S, Aeschlimann A, Schwyzer HK, Simmen BR. Responsiveness of six outcome assessment instruments in total shoulder arthroplasty. Arthritis Rheum 2008;59:391–8.
8. Angst F, Goldhahn J, Drerup S, Flury M, Schwyzer HK, Simmen BR. How sharp is the short QuickDASH? A refined content and validity analysis of the short form of the disabilities of the shoulder, arm and hand questionnaire in the strata of symptoms and function and specific joint conditions. Qual Life Res 2009;18:1043–51.
9. Angst F, Goldhahn J, Pap G, Mannion AF, Roach KE, Siebertz D, Drerup S, Schwyzer HK, Simmen BR. Cross-cultural adaptation, reliability and validity of the German Shoulder Pain and Disability Index (SPADI). Rheumatology (Oxford) 2007;46:87–92.
10. Angst F, Pap G, Mannion AF, Herren DB, Aeschlimann A, Schwyzer HK, Simmen BR. Comprehensive assessment of clinical outcome and quality of life after total shoulder arthroplasty: usefulness and validity of subjective outcome measures. Arthritis Rheum 2004;51:819–28.
11. Basaran S, Guzel R, Seydaoglu G, Guler-Uysal F. Validity, reliability, and comparison of the WOMAC osteoarthritis index and Lequesne algofunctional index in Turkish patients with hip or knee osteoarthritis. Clin Rheumatol 2010;29:749–56.
12. Beaton D, Richards RR. Assessing the reliability and responsiveness of 5 shoulder questionnaires. J Shoulder Elbow Surg 1998;7:565–72.
13. Beaton DE, Kennedy CA. Beyond return to work: testing a measure of at-work disability in workers with musculoskeletal pain. Qual Life Res 2005;14:1869–79.

14. Beaton DE, Wright JG, Katz JN. Development of the QuickDASH: comparison of three item-reduction approaches. J Bone Joint Surg Am 2005;87:1038–46.
15. Bellamy N. WOMAC Osteoarthritis Index User Guide IV; 2010.
16. Bellamy N. WOMAC Osteoarthritis Index, 2014. Accessed September 3, 2015, at http://womac.org/womac/index.htm.
17. Bellamy N, Campbell J, Haraoui B, Buchbinder R, Hobby K, Roth JH, MacDermid JC. Dimensionality and clinical importance of pain and disability in hand osteoarthritis: development of the Australian/Canadian (AUSCAN) Osteoarthritis Hand Index. Osteoarthritis Cartilage 2002;10:855–62.
18. Bennett MI, Smith BH, Torrance N, Potter J. The S-LANSS score for identifying pain of predominantly neuropathic origin: validation for use in clinical and postal research. J Pain 2005;6:149–58.
19. Bijur PE, Silver W, Gallagher EJ. Reliability of the visual analog scale for measurement of acute pain. Acad Emerg Med 2001;8:1153–57.
20. Boardman DL, Dorey F, Thomas BJ, Lieberman JR. The accuracy of assessing total hip arthroplasty outcomes: a prospective correlation study of walking ability and 2 validated measurement devices. J Arthroplasty 2000;15:200–4.
21. Bond M, Davis A, Lohmander S, Hawker G. Responsiveness of the OARSI-OMERACT osteoarthritis pain and function measures. Osteoarthritis Cartilage 2012;20:541–7.
22. Boonstra AM, Schiphorst Preuper HR, Balk GA, Stewart RE. Cut-off points for mild, moderate, and severe pain on the visual analogue scale for pain in patients with chronic musculoskeletal pain. Pain 2014;155:2545–50.
23. Burckhardt CS, Bjelle A. A Swedish version of the short-form McGill Pain Questionnaire. Scand J Rheumatol 1994;23:77–81.
24. Cappelleri JC, Bienen EJ, Koduru V, Sadosky A. Measurement properties of painDETECT by average pain severity. Clinicoecon Outcomes Res 2014;6:497–504.
25. Cappelleri JC, Koduru V, Bienen EJ, Sadosky A. A cross-sectional study examining the psychometric properties of the painDETECT measure in neuropathic pain. J Pain Res 2015;8:159–67.
26. Collins SL, Moore RA, McQuay HJ. The visual analogue pain intensity scale: what is moderate pain in millimetres? Pain 1997;72:95–7.
27. Davis AM, Lohmander LS, Wong R, Venkataramanan V, Hawker GA. Evaluating the responsiveness of the ICOAP following hip or knee replacement. Osteoarthritis Cartilage 2010;18:1043–45.
28. Davis AM, Perruccio AV, Canizares M, Hawker GA, Roos EM, Maillefert JF, Lohmander LS. Comparative, validity and responsiveness of the HOOS-PS and KOOS-PS to the WOMAC physical function subscale in total joint replacement for osteoarthritis. Osteoarthritis Cartilage 2009;17:843–7.
29. Davison MJ, Ioannidis G, Maly MR, Adachi JD, Beattie KA. Intermittent and constant pain and physical function or performance in men and women with knee osteoarthritis: data from the osteoarthritis initiative. Clinical Rheumatol 2016;35:371–9.
30. Downie WW, Leatham PA, Rhind VM, Wright V, Branco JA, Anderson JA. Studies with pain rating scales. Ann Rheum Dis 1978;37:378–381.

31. Dworkin RH, Turk DC, Farrar JT, Haythornthwaite JA, Jensen MP, Katz NP, Kerns RD, Stucki G, Allen RR, Bellamy N, et al. Core outcome measures for chronic pain clinical trials: IMMPACT recommendations. Pain 2005;113:9–19.
32. Ekeberg OM, Bautz-Holter E, Keller A, Tveita EK, Juel NG, Brox JI. A questionnaire found disease-specific WORC index is not more responsive than SPADI and OSS in rotator cuff disease. J Clin Epidemiol 2010;63:575–84.
33. Escobar A, Quintana JM, Bilbao A, Arostegui I, Lafuente I, Vidaurreta I. Responsiveness and clinically important differences for the WOMAC and SF-36 after total knee replacement. Osteoarthritis Cartilage 2007;15:273–80.
34. Escobar A, Quintana JM, Bilbao A, Azkarate J, Guenaga JI. Validation of the Spanish version of the WOMAC questionnaire for patients with hip or knee osteoarthritis. Western Ontario and McMaster Universities Osteoarthritis Index. Clin Rheumatol 2002;21:466–71.
35. Farrar JT, Young JP Jr, LaMoreaux L, Werth JL, Poole RM. Clinical importance of changes in chronic pain intensity measured on an 11-point numerical pain rating scale. Pain 2001;94:149–58.
36. Ferraz MB, Quaresma MR, Aquino LR, Atra E, Tugwell P, Goldsmith CH. Reliability of pain scales in the assessment of literate and illiterate patients with rheumatoid arthritis. J Rheumatol 1990;17:1022–24.
37. Finch E, Walsh M, Thomas SG, Woodhouse LJ. Functional ability perceived by individuals following total knee arthroplasty compared to age-matched individuals without knee disability. J Orthop Sports Phys Ther 1998;27:255–63.
38. Franchignoni F, Vercelli S, Giordano A, Sartorio F, Bravini E, Ferriero G. Minimal clinically important difference of the disabilities of the arm, shoulder and hand outcome measure (DASH) and its shortened version (QuickDASH). J Orthop Sports Phys Ther 2014;44:30–9.
39. Freynhagen R, Baron R, Gockel U, Tolle TR. painDETECT: a new screening questionnaire to identify neuropathic components in patients with back pain. Curr Med Res Opin 2006;22:1911–20.
40. Gandhi R, Tsvetkov D, Dhottar H, Davey JR, Mahomed NN. Quantifying the pain experience in hip and knee osteoarthritis. Pain Res Manag 2010;15:224–8.
41. Gill SD, de Morton NA, Mc Burney H. An investigation of the validity of six measures of physical function in people awaiting joint replacement surgery of the hip or knee. Clin Rehabil 2012;26:945–51.
42. Goncalves RS, Meireles AC, Gil JN, Cavalheiro LM, Rosado JO, Cabri J. Responsiveness of intermittent and constant osteoarthritis pain (ICOAP) after physical therapy for knee osteoarthritis. Osteoarthritis Cartilage 2012;20:1116–9.
43. Grafton KV, Foster NE, Wright CC. Test-retest reliability of the Short-Form McGill Pain Questionnaire: assessment of intraclass correlation coefficients and limits of agreement in patients with osteoarthritis. Clin J Pain 2005;21:73–82.
44. Gummesson C, Ward MM, Atroshi I. The shortened disabilities of the arm, shoulder and hand questionnaire (QuickDASH): validity and reliability based on responses within the full-length DASH. BMC Musculoskelet Disord 2006; 7:44.
45. Hawker G, Davis A, French M, Cibere J, Jordan J, March L, Suarez-Almazor M, Katz J, Dieppe P. Development and preliminary psychometric testing of a new

OA pain measure—an OARSI/OMERACT initiative. Osteoarthritis Cartilage 2008;16:409–14.
46. Hawker GA, Mian S, Kendzerska T, French M. Measures of adult pain: Visual Analog Scale for Pain (VAS Pain), Numeric Rating Scale for Pain (NRS Pain), McGill Pain Questionnaire (MPQ), Short-Form McGill Pain Questionnaire (SF-MPQ), Chronic Pain Grade Scale (CPGS), Short Form-36 Bodily Pain Scale (SF-36 BPS), and Measure of Intermittent and Constant Osteoarthritis Pain (ICOAP). Arthritis Care Res (Hoboken) 2011;63:S240–52.
47. Heald SL, Riddle DL, Lamb RL. The shoulder pain and disability index: the construct validity and responsiveness of a region-specific disability measure. Phys Ther 1997;77:1079–89.
48. Institute for Work and Health. The DASH Outcome Measure. 2015. Accessed at http://dash.iwh.on.ca.
49. Jensen MP, Chen C, Brugger AM. Interpretation of visual analog scale ratings and change scores: a reanalysis of two clinical trials of postoperative pain. J Pain 2003;4:407–14.
50. Jensen MP, Karoly P, Braver S. The measurement of clinical pain intensity: a comparison of six methods. Pain 1986;27:117–26.
51. Johanson NA, Liang MH, Daltroy L, Rudicel S, Richmond J. American Academy of Orthopaedic Surgeons lower limb outcomes assessment instruments. Reliability, validity, and sensitivity to change. J Bone Joint Surg Am 2004;86-A:902–9.
52. Kessler S, Grammozis A, Gunther KP, Kirschner S. The intermittent and constant pain score (ICOAP)—a questionnaire to assess pain in patients with gonarthritis. Zeitschrift fur Orthopadie und Unfallchirurgie 2011;149:22–6.
53. Konstantinidis GA, Aletras VH, Kanakari KA, Natsis K, Bellamy N, Niakas D. Comparative validation of the WOMAC osteoarthritis and Lequesne algofunctional indices in Greek patients with hip or knee osteoarthritis. Qual Life Res 2014;23:539–48.
54. Macdermid JC, Khadilkar L, Birmingham TB, Athwal GS. Validity of the QuickDASH in patients with shoulder-related disorders undergoing surgery. J Orthop Sports Phys Ther 2015;45:25–36.
55. Maska L, Anderson J, Michaud K. Measures of functional status and quality of life in rheumatoid arthritis: Health Assessment Questionnaire Disability Index (HAQ), Modified Health Assessment Questionnaire (MHAQ), Multidimensional Health Assessment Questionnaire (MDHAQ), Health Assessment Questionnaire II (HAQ-II), Improved Health Assessment Questionnaire (Improved HAQ), and Rheumatoid Arthritis Quality of Life (RAQoL). Arthritis Care Res (Hoboken) 2011;63:S4–13.
56. Mathieson S, Lin C. painDETECT questionnaire. J Physiother 2013;59:211.
57. McCormack HM, Horne DJ, Sheather S. Clinical applications of visual analogue scales: a critical review. Psychol Med 1988;18:1007–19.
58. Melzack R. The short-form McGill Pain Questionnaire. Pain 1987;30:191–7.
59. Michener LA, Snyder AR, Leggin BG. Responsiveness of the numeric pain rating scale in patients with shoulder pain and the effect of surgical status. J Sport Rehabil 2011;20:115–28.

60. Mintken PE, Glynn P, Cleland JA. Psychometric properties of the shortened disabilities of the Arm, Shoulder, and Hand Questionnaire (QuickDASH) and Numeric Pain Rating Scale in patients with shoulder pain. J Shoulder Elbow Surg 2009;18:920–6.
61. Moreton BJ, Tew V, das Nair R, Wheeler M, Walsh DA, Lincoln NB. Pain phenotype in patients with knee osteoarthritis: classification and measurement properties of painDETECT and self-report Leeds assessment of neuropathic symptoms and signs scale in a cross-sectional study. Arthritis Care Res (Hoboken) 2015;67:519–28.
62. Ornetti P, Dougados M, Paternotte S, Logeart I, Gossec L. Validation of a numerical rating scale to assess functional impairment in hip and knee osteoarthritis: comparison with the WOMAC function scale. Ann Rheum Dis 2011;70:740–6.
63. Riley SP, Cote MP, Swanson B, Tafuto V, Sizer PS, Brismee JM. The Shoulder Pain and Disability Index: is it sensitive and responsive to immediate change? Man Ther 2015;20:494–8.
64. Roach KE, Budiman-Mak E, Songsiridej N, Lertratanakul Y. Development of a shoulder pain and disability index. Arthritis Care Res 1991;4:143–9.
65. Robbins SM, Rastogi R, Howard J, Rosedale R. Comparison of measurement properties of the P4 pain scale and disease specific pain measures in patients with knee osteoarthritis. Osteoarthritis Cartilage 2014;22:805–12.
66. Rodriguez CS. Pain measurement in the elderly: a review. Pain Manag Nurs 2001;2:38–46.
67. Roy JS, MacDermid JC, Amick BC 3rd, Shannon HS, McMurtry R, Roth JH, Grewal R, Tang K, Beaton D. Validity and responsiveness of presenteeism scales in chronic work-related upper-extremity disorders. Phys Ther 2011;91:254–66.
68. Roy JS, MacDermid JC, Woodhouse LJ. Measuring shoulder function: a systematic review of four questionnaires. Arthritis Rheum 2009;61:623–32.
69. Schmitt JS, Di Fabio RP. Reliable change and minimum important difference (MID) proportions facilitated group responsiveness comparisons using individual threshold criteria. J Clin Epidemiol 2004;57:1008–18.
70. Scott J, Huskisson EC. Graphic representation of pain. Pain 1976;2:175–84.
71. Singh JA, Luo R, Landon GC, Suarez-Almazor M. Reliability and clinically important improvement thresholds for osteoarthritis pain and function scales: a multicenter study. J Rheumatol 2014;41:509–15.
72. Soderman P, Malchau H. Validity and reliability of Swedish WOMAC osteoarthritis index: a self-administered disease-specific questionnaire (WOMAC) versus generic instruments (SF-36 and NHP). Acta Orthop Scand 2000;71:39–46.
73. Staples MP, Forbes A, Green S, Buchbinder R. Shoulder-specific disability measures showed acceptable construct validity and responsiveness. J Clin Epidemiol 2010;63:163–70.
74. Strand LI, Ljunggren AE, Bogen B, Ask T, Johnsen TB. The Short-Form McGill Pain Questionnaire as an outcome measure: test-retest reliability and responsiveness to change. Eur J Pain 2008;12:917–25.
75. Tampin B, Briffa NK, Goucke R, Slater H. Identification of neuropathic pain in patients with neck/upper limb pain: application of a grading system and screening tools. Pain 2013;154:2813–22.

76. Tashjian RZ, Deloach J, Porucznik CA, Powell AP. Minimal clinically important differences (MCID) and patient acceptable symptomatic state (PASS) for visual analog scales (VAS) measuring pain in patients treated for rotator cuff disease. J Shoulder Elbow Surg 2009;18:927–32.
77. Tubach F, Ravaud P, Baron G, Falissard B, Logeart I, Bellamy N, Bombardier C, Felson D, Hochberg M, van der Heijde D, Dougados M. Evaluation of clinically relevant changes in patient reported outcomes in knee and hip osteoarthritis: the minimal clinically important improvement. Ann Rheum Dis 2005;64:29–33.
78. Tveita EK, Ekeberg OM, Juel NG, Bautz-Holter E. Responsiveness of the shoulder pain and disability index in patients with adhesive capsulitis. BMC Musculoskelet Disord 2008;9:161.
79. Wigler I, Neumann L, Yaron M. Validation study of a Hebrew version of WOMAC in patients with osteoarthritis of the knee. Clin Rheumatol 1999;18:402–5.
80. Williams JW Jr, Holleman DR Jr, Simel DL. Measuring shoulder function with the Shoulder Pain and Disability Index. J Rheumatol 1995;22:727–32.
81. Wolfe F, Michaud K, Pincus T. Development and validation of the health assessment questionnaire II: a revised version of the health assessment questionnaire. Arthritis Rheum 2004;50:3296–305.
82. Wright JG, Young NL. A comparison of different indices of responsiveness. J Clin Epidemiol 1997;50:239–46.

CHAPTER 8

# Assessing Joint Pain Experimentally in Humans

*Lars Arendt-Nielsen and Kristian Kjær Petersen*

In the development process of new and better pharmacological and nonpharmacological treatment regimens for chronic joint pain (e.g., osteoarthritis [OA]), it is important to have tools available for assessing the underlying peripheral and central pain mechanisms. Likewise, it is important to have diagnostic tools available for stratifying and subgrouping patients for the purpose of individualized management.

Simple pain ratings and questionnaires do not allow differentiating between the different pain mechanisms involved such as local and generalized hyperalgesia, and peripheral versus central pain mechanisms.

A higher degree of general sensitization in OA has been shown to be related to higher levels of pain [7, 29], disability, poorer quality of life [41], worse spreading sensitization [78], poorer outcome after total joint replacement surgery [59, 89], and higher concentration of proinflammatory cytokines [55]. It seems of importance to have tools available to quantify the degree of sensitization in OA and possible use of this in the management for, for example, preventing further development of the pain chronification process [17].

The lack of association between the individual OA patient's pain intensity and objective radiological findings [21, 36, 63, 79] and the existence of specific OA subgroups [3, 4, 29] is strong indications that pain facilitatory or inhibitory mechanisms are involved. It is not fully understood why some patients continue to have chronic pain after joint replacement and why others are pain free, but emerging evidence suggests that central pain mechanisms can be involved [14, 70, 71, 89].

Human quantitative experimental pain assessment tools (named mechanism-based pain biomarkers or quantitative sensory testing [QST]) have in recent years been substantially developed to provide a technological platform for assessing pain in musculoskeletal conditions. The experimental techniques may provide quantitative information about gain of function and loss of function in the sensitivity of the pain system and specific pain mechanisms.

Previously, the technological approaches had predominantly been developed for and applied in the area of neuropathic pain where cutaneous manifestations (e.g., tactile hyperalgesia, brush-evoked allodynia, thermal hyperalgesia) were assessed. In musculoskeletal conditions and specifically in joint pain, it is more complicated to stimulate directly and selectively the structures involved and assess their sensitivity.

This chapter will focus on test methods developed for assessing quantitatively how specific pain reactions or mechanisms are altered in patients with joint pain and in particular OA as most studies have been published in this area. Such a mechanism-based assessment approach may help translating the knowledge obtained in animal studies and provide a better understanding of the impact of joint pain on the human nervous system.

## THE CONCEPT OF HUMAN EXPERIMENTAL PAIN ASSESSMENT

Application of QST technologies for assessing joint pain involves a variety of painful stimulus modalities and assessment methods providing different information about pain transduction, transmission, and perception.

The evoked response can be assessed by psychophysical methods (thresholds, stimulus–response functions), electrophysiological responses (e.g., evoked potentials), or imaging (e.g., fMRI). Such measures can be associated with the clinical examinations (e.g., X-ray, MRI), clinical pain assessments (pain intensity, quality, duration, temporal/spatial distributions), and/or biochemical markers in serum, synovial fluid, or cerebrospinal fluid.

It has become obvious that the heterogeneity among knee OA patients has an impact on treatment outcome [39, 48].

In a sample of 52 OA patients, three different groups were found based on the presence of inflammatory infiltrates in the synovial fluid: 43% of them had no inflammatory infiltrates, 50% had low-grade inflammatory infiltrates, and 7% had high inflammatory infiltrates [68]. In a study combining experimental pain biomarkers, clinical assessments, and serological markers, three distinct groups of OA patients were identified [24].

The multidimensional nature of joint pain cannot be assessed in details based on a single method but needs a more comprehensive approach and combination of methods. The combination of experimental/clinical pain measures and biochemical markers provide new opportunity to establish individual profiles of patients, which in the future may be the basis for individualized treatment and for more advanced clinical trials on new treatments [22, 24, 82]. Furthermore, the psychological profiles of individual patients should also be considered as part of the profiling [18].

## EXPERIMENTAL PAIN ASSESSMENT TOOLS

The psychophysical determinations can be divided into stimulus-dependent and response-dependent methods. The stimulus-dependent methods are based on adjustment of the stimulus intensity until pain detection or tolerance threshold is reached. The response-dependent methods rely on pain intensity ratings to a series of fixed stimulus intensities and a score to each stimulus (e.g., visual analog scale [VAS]). The stimulus intensity is normally varied in the interval between pain detection and pain tolerance.

Predominantly, four stimulus modalities have proven to be useful for assessing the consequences of OA on pain sensitivity: pressure pain thresholds, thermal thresholds, cold pressor–evoked pain, and pinprick. In knee OA, the sites tested are normally around the knee (patella, medial and lateral aspects of the knee), muscles around the knee (quadriceps and tibialis anterior), and sites away from the knee (forearm, finger, and trapezium) for assessing both the localized and the generalized pain hypersensitivity.

A few studies have examined the reliability of experimental pain assessment in OA [85, 87] and found good reliability.

In general, OA patients are more sensitive to various painful stimuli as compared with age-matched controls [55], with 70% of knee OA patients having at least one somatosensory abnormality [86].

Several recent meta-analysis [30, 80] and reviews [9, 57] have been published, providing comprehensive analysis of all relevant sensory tests investigated in OA.

When comparing men and women with symptomatic knee OA, it seems women show a greater degree of sensitization to the various experimental pain stimuli (lower heat, cold, pressure thresholds/tolerances, greater temporal summation of pain) as compared with men [12].

## Pressure Stimulation

Only one human study has been published in which intra-articular pressure has been applied [23]. Externally applied pressure is used in many studies, but it could be discussed if any intra-articular structures are actually activated as pain can likewise be evoked from patients after total knee replacement [77], indicating that the extra-articular structures (muscles, ligaments, skin) are involved.

Pressure pain is found as a reliable technique for assessing sensitivity in OA [62, 87], and many studies have shown lower pressure pain thresholds in OA when assessed around the affected knee joint [80], with a positive association to the clinical pain intensity [3, 51].

Generally, one can find a significant correlation between pressure pain sensitivity and symptom severity [34, 64], but Skou et al. [77] found no relationship between pressure pain and clinical pain intensity most likely because the study was not powered for investigating this relationship.

Pressure pain assessment performed with a handheld algometer provides reliable responses [43]. More recently, more advanced computer-controlled pressure stimulation has further improved the reliability as experimenter bias (and interobserver variability) can be removed. This technique also allows a reliable way to evoked stimulus–response functions and temporal summation of pressure pain [65].

If pressure pain thresholds are determined from various locations over the knee, a topographical pain sensitivity map can be constructed [7]. This can likewise be done for a variety of other musculoskeletal structures [15] and disorders [28].

In OA, the pressure pain sensitivity maps have provided new opportunities to profile individual patients with different degrees of pain, joint damage, and synovitis. Fig. 8-1 shows examples of individual pressure sensitivity maps.

As handheld or computer-controlled pressure algometer activates a small volume of tissue, a computer-controlled cuff algometry technique has been developed. The pain threshold or the pain intensity related to standardized inflations (stimulus–response curves) of a tourniquet applied around an extremity can be established [44]. The cuff algometry cannot be applied directly to a joint for assessing local hyperalgesia in OA patients but to extremities for assessing the generalized pain hypersensitivity [3] and have been shown to be reliable for measurements of widespread hyperalgesia and temporal summation [33], of which temporal summation can be used to predict the outcome after knee replacement [70].

## Thermal Stimulation

Although thermal stimulation activates the cutaneous nociceptors, there are studies showing changes in thermal sensitivity in OA. Most data indicating reduced sensitivity [27, 86] depend on the location of assessment [51]. In other studies, no significant changes are found in thermal thresholds [35, 72].

Four studies have compared heat pain thresholds in knee OA patients with healthy controls [46, 55, 86, 88]. Lee et al. [55] found increased pain responses to a 49° and 51° thermal pulses in OA patients.

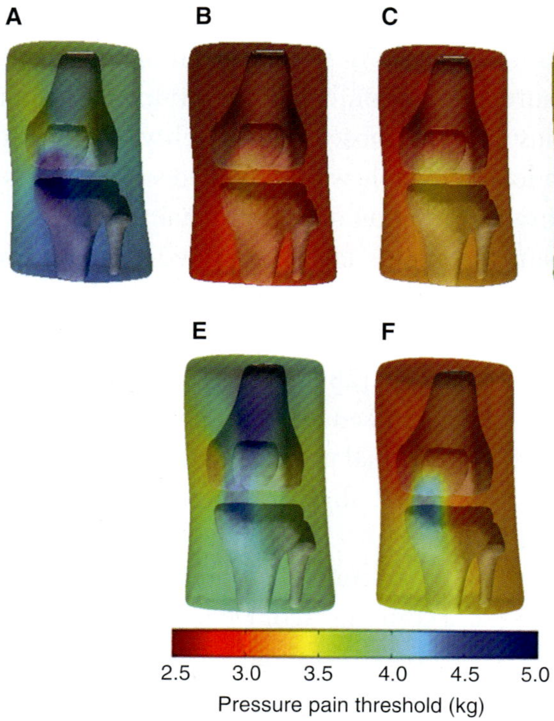


**FIGURE 8-1** Pressure pain sensitivity maps for different individual OA pain patients and from a control volunteer. The colors indicate the pressure pain threshold in kPa where blue represents high thresholds and red low threshold (hyperalgesia). The map is constructed based on 10 individual threshold assessments around the knee, and the map is constructed based on interpolation between the individual thresholds. The map structure is extracted from the knee surface determined on basis of MRI scans. **A:** The sensitivity map from a control volunteers where the threshold is generally high. **B:** OA patients with high clinical pain intensity. **C:** OA patient with joint with minimal damage (KL2) but high pain. **D:** OA patient with severe joint damage (KL4) but minimal clinical pain. **E:** OA patients with low degree of synovitis. **F:** OA patients with high degree of synovitis.

A meta-analysis showed no local sensitivity changes over the knee, but at remote locations, heat hyperalgesia can be detected [30]. Finan et al. [29] found that a specific knee OA group with high pain intensity/low disease severity showed stronger responses to heat pain in the forearm than other knee OA groups.

Assessment of cold hyperalgesia has been inconclusive in OA [67], and some found hypoesthesia to cold detection thresholds [37]. Finan et al. [29] found no differences in the cold pressor pain response.

### Pinprick Stimulation

Studies have revealed tactile hypoesthesia [38]. Harden and coworkers [37] found that most OA patients had abnormalities to pinprick (41% were hyperalgesic and 27% were hypoesthetic), and in other studies, it seems that for increased stimulus intensities pinprick hyperalgesia can be found in OA patients as compared with controls [35]. This is supported by other groups [46].

Pinprick hyperalgesia [72] is associated with the degree on OA pain.

## MECHANISTIC ASSESSMENT OF JOINT PAIN

From preclinical OA model studies, it is well known that a variety of peripheral and central pain mechanisms may be modulated, and the attempt is to translate those findings into human OA patients to acquire more mechanistic information [5]. However, recordings from dorsal horn neurons are not possible; so other more indirect measures of sensitization have to be utilized in humans [9]. In general, the pain hypersensitivity is most pronounced in OA patients with the strongest pain [46] and the longest pain duration [3]. Three mechanisms will briefly be addressed here.

### Local versus Widespread Hyperalgesia

Assessing pain thresholds from the knee area versus a remote area will provide information about the extrasegmental spreading of sensitization. It has consistently across different research groups [7, 24, 34, 40, 50, 55, 86] been shown that spreading sensitization is a feature in OA patients, which most likely depends on the clinical pain intensity and pain duration [9].

It has recently been shown that preoperative widespread hyperalgesia is being linked to the development of chronic postoperative pain following total joint replacement [70, 89].

As such, it is evident that joint pain in humans also has a significant impact on the entire nervous system, and this should be taken into consideration in management and in the development of new therapeutics.

## Temporal Summation

Temporal summation is a measure for central integrative mechanisms induced by sequence of stimuli with the same intensity. Temporal summation mimics the initial phase of the windup process, which has been measured in the dorsal horn in animal studies. Healthy controls feel the tenth stimulus as slightly more painful than the first, whereas sensitized OA patients feel a large pain difference [9]. Preoperative temporal summation has been shown to predict the development of chronic postoperative pain following total knee replacement surgery [70].

Temporal summation can be evoked by a variety of stimuli such as tactile pinprick, pressure, heat, and electrical pulses.

For simple bedside testing, temporal summation evoked by repeated mechanical punctate pain stimuli has been used in OA [5, 18, 29], and the summation has shown association with the pain severity but not the radiographic severity [64]. The subgroup of OA patients with high knee pain and low knee radiographic grade showed more facilitated temporal summation to punctate pain stimuli than the other groups [29]. Repeated punctuate stimuli seem to be a sensitive model for assessing facilitated central integration in OA.

Studies using repeated thermal stimuli are less conclusive, as two studies have shown subgroup differences when assessed from the forearm [29] and at the knee [18]. One study did not show any differences [46].

Repeated pressure stimuli using computer-controlled algometry or cuff algometry have shown facilitated temporal summation when assessed from the knee and from arm/leg with an association to pain severity and duration but not radiographic severity [3, 7, 77].

Facilitated temporal summation has been found in patients with pain after total knee replacement as compared with those who became pain free [76]. In addition, those patients with chronic pain after knee replacement showed even more facilitated summation as compared with OA patients prior to surgery [78].

### Conditioning Pain Modulation

In recent years, there has been increased focus on the function of the descending pathways in humans. Animal studies have shown that both descending facilitation and inhibition have an impact on the entire neuroaxis, explaining one aspect of generalized widespread hyperalgesia. In humans, we can only assess the net sum of the descending drive in the two pathways, and the general finding is that in chronic pain patients, the potency of the pain inhibition is impaired [10, 56] and this is particularly evident in patients with musculoskeletal disorders [19].

A number of studies have found significant impaired conditioning pain modulation (CPM) in OA with an association to both pain intensity and pain duration [3, 7, 24, 49] and found that the CPM is restored in patients after knee replacement whereby the patients become pain free [34]. OA patients with chronic pain after knee replacement continue to have impaired descending control [77].

Finan et al. [29] found no difference in CPM potency between different OA subgroups, and King et al. [46] found no differences between OA patients and controls.

Studies have challenged reliability of CPM assessment because of the large inter- and intraindividual variation [66], and various attempts have been made to refine the technique [16]. Recently, the cuff algometry technique has been applied in which one cuff delivers the conditioning stimulus and another cuff delivers the test stimulus [33, 70].

## BIOCHEMICAL ASSESSMENT TOOLS

As there are weak associations between macroscopic changes of the joint and the clinical/experimental pain manifestations, attempt has been made to associate biochemical markers with the pain biomarkers. It has been established that synovitis and bone remodeling biomarkers contribute to the joint pain [42].

The synovial membrane consists of type I and III collagen [26, 58]. During inflammation, the synovial membrane undergoes fibrogenesis, while markers of type I or III collagen turnover could reflect the severity of synovitis. Several studies have shown increased levels of matrix metalloproteinase (MMP)-derived degradation products of type I and type III collagen (C1M and C3M) in rheumatoid arthritis, and C1M is increased in patients with end-stage OA [74]. C1M is not a biomarker of bone degradation as the fragment generated by MMPs is further degraded by cathepsin K, the most abundant protease in bone.

The synovial membrane is densely packed with nociceptive fibers [25, 32], and inflammation and degeneration could alter pain perception from the joint [69, 84]. A MMP-derived fragment of type II collagen, C2M, reflects cartilage degradation and is elevated in patients with radiographic OA [13].

Biomarkers of inflammation are relevant as well, and C-reactive protein (CRP) is elevated in OA patient and CRP levels seem to correlate with pressure pain thresholds [55], indicating that inflammation could play a role in sensitization. High-sensitive CRP (hsCRP) is elevated in the later stages of OA compared with earlier stages [74] and is a sensitive biomarker of acute and systemic inflammation [53], whereas the MMP-derived fragment of CRP (CRPM) seems to be a sensitive marker of local tissue inflammation [75].

So far, very limited associations have been found between joint-related biomarkers and pain reactions. In a comprehensive OA study, attempt was made to associate all the above-mentioned markers with the experimental pain biomarkers, and the only consistent finding was associations between CPM and temporal summation and hsCRP [4, 24]. Similarly, Lee et al. [55] found an association between CRP levels and pressure pain thresholds assessed from nonknee sites.

Besides joint-related biomarkers, attempts have been made to associate neuroinflammatory markers with experimental pain biomarkers.

In knee OA patients and matched controls, pro- (IL-6, IL-8, and tumor necrosis factor alpha [TNF-α]) and anti-inflammatory (IL-10) cytokines were correlated with the pressure pain threshold, and only the TNF-α level was found to be correlated [40].

A single study has reported that higher preoperative levels of TNF-α, MMP-13, and IL-6 in the synovial fluid of OA patients were associated with a smaller improvement in pain 2 years after total knee replacement [31].

## PATIENT PROFILING

Profiling of specific patient populations is most developed in the area of neuropathic pain, and less has been done in the area of musculoskeletal pain and in particular joint pain.

It is, however, evident that a variety of experimental pain markers are attenuated in patients with OA and that they reflect changes in nociceptive processing in peripheral and central nervous structures, depending on pain severity and duration [9]. Furthermore, there may be serological markers, such as the degradation marker CTX-II, that could as well be indicative for disease status and possible disease progression [20]. A combination of selected biomarkers can include assessment of spreading sensitization by pressure pain thresholds, facilitated temporal summation, impaired descending modulation, and hsCRP as they seem specifically adequate for inclusion in a sensitization index [3, 24] could be a valuable tool for profiling and subgrouping joint pain patients. A more comprehensive approach should also include the most relevant clinical pain parameters (Western Ontario and McMaster Universities Osteoarthritis Index, PainDETECT) and psychological features such as catastrophizing.

Further developments in this field of profiling joint pain patients should (1) focus on development of simple user-independent bedside pain assessment tools, (2) define normative ranges and risk zones/profiles (Fig. 8-2), and (3) link the profiles to management and prevention strategies.

Pain profiling in joint pain has three obvious applications as described below.

### Diagnostic Purpose for Individualized Treatment

Today, the treatment options for joint management are far from being individualized, and various treatment guidelines have been published. Those guidelines are for obvious reasons not based on a mechanistic approach in which the treatment is tailored to pain mechanism. The challenge in future research is to start linking the pain assessment date with drug effects. Today, the treatment options are limited to topicals,

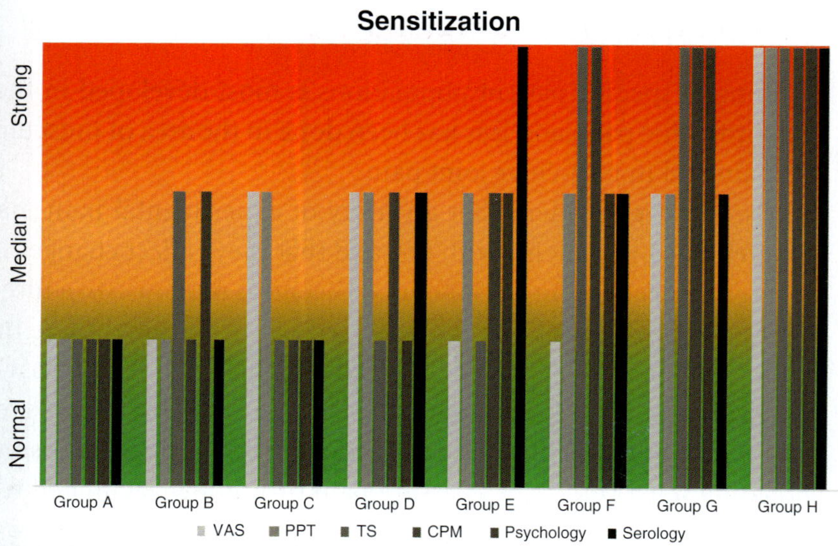


**FIGURE 8-2** A schematic figure showing a theoretical outcome of measures from eight different groups, ranging from controls (group A) to a severe OA patients (group H) with a strong degree of sensitization for all the measures assessed. The bars represent the clinical pain intensity score (VAS), the pressure pain threshold (PPT), temporal summation (TS), descending pain modulation (CPM), a psychological score (e.g., catastrophizing), and a serological marker (e.g., hsCRP). Each measures, as a single representative of sensitization, can range from normal (**green area**) via moderate (**orange**) to strong (**red**). The more measures showing strong sensitization, the more dramatically impacted the pain system is, and hence combination of peripherally and centrally acting drugs are needed and the patients may be more vulnerable for developing chronic pain after joint surgery.

nonsteroidal anti-inflammatory drugs, cyclooxygenase-II inhibitors, acetaminophen plus/minus codeine and for the more severe pain cases gabapentinoids, antidepressants, and in rare cases opioids like oxycodone, tramadol, and tapentadol may be options for short-term use as the marginal effect is counteracted by unwanted side effects. Alternative treatments such as viscosupplementation (e.g., hyaluronic acid) [73], glucosamine, and chondroitin [83] have no proven long-term effect in OA. In recent years, exercise has proven its role in OA and now has been included in many guidelines [54, 81], but so far no studies have investigated which subgroups of patients benefit most from such exercise programs.

## Predicting Outcome of Joint Replacement

The incidence of total knee replacements is expected to increase in the United States by almost 700% toward 2030 [52], and the procedure is associated with risk of adverse events. Around 20% undergoing knee replacement experience only small or no improvements in pain [14], and more knee pain is known to be related to lower patient satisfaction [1].

Chronic postoperative pain after knee replacement or revision surgery is a substantial clinical problem, known to affect between 5% and 85% of patients [45, 60, 71]. The role of peripheral and widespread sensitizations as predictors for development of chronic postoperative pain after joint replacement or revision surgery has recently been suggested [70, 77, 78], and more studies in the future will determine which of the pain biomarkers are the best predictors. This topic is addressed in detail in Chapter 11.

## Drug Development

Development of new drugs for OA pain is a major challenge as the costs for developing new compounds steadily increase and the number of new analgesics approved is very low. Furthermore, the widespread pain sensitization component is difficult to manage without unwanted side effects, and hence, the development goes in the direction of peripherally restricted compounds, damping the peripheral drive, and hence the central consequences [2]. Hence, there is a need to optimize the drug development process, and advanced technology platforms of translational, mechanism-based human pain biomarkers are promising tools in this optimization process [6, 8]. Over five decades (1960–2009) of drug development for treatment of pain, 39 drugs have been specifically developed as analgesics, and 20 drugs have been developed for nonpain indications but have shown to be effective in pain [47]. However, many compounds have failed in OA despite good analgesic effects in a variety of animal OA models, indicating that the current animal models do not mimic the mechanisms of OA pain in humans [5]. In general, this lack of efficacy contributes to 51% of Phase 2 trial failures [11].

A review by Pfizer researchers summarized the benefits of predictive biomarkers in drug development [61]. The analysis was performed on data from Phase 2 decisions for 44 programs at Pfizer. Not only were most failures caused by a lack of efficacy, but also, in several cases (43%), it was not possible to conclude whether the mechanism had been adequately tested. A key finding was that an integrated understanding of the fundamental mechanistic and pharmacokinetic/pharmacodynamic principles of exposure at the site of action, target binding, and expression of functional pharmacological activity determined the likelihood of candidate survival in Phase 2 trials and improved the chance of progression to Phase 3. They referred to an example in which a dopamine D3 receptor agonist showed a positive effect in the rat monosodium iodoacetate (OA model) model. A randomized, double-blind, placebo, and active-controlled crossover study was conducted in OA, showing no beneficial effect.

A mechanistic drug profiling approach to characterize analgesic and antihyperalgesic actions is not limited to proof-of-concept studies of new compounds under development but can also be utilized for profiling existing analgesics with action mechanisms that are not fully known. Mechanism-based proof-of-concept Phase 1b or 2a trials if positive may be predictive for which subgroups of OA patients may benefit, and hence, the later larger clinical trials can be enriched and thus optimized. Drug profiling coupled with comprehensive patient profiling using mechanistic pain biomarkers seems to be the way to optimize analgesic drug development for joint pain conditions in the future.

## CONCLUSIONS

The status of the nociceptors in a damaged joint and its surroundings cannot be measured directly, but a variety of quantitative experimental pain assessment tools have been developed to provide some information about the mechanisms underlying joint pain in humans.

Local and spreading sensitization, central temporal integration, and descending pain modulation are features that can be assessed and used for profiling patients.

It is evident that there exist subgroups of patients with joint pain, in particular OA, and quantitative pain assessment tools can help stratification of patients and hence be used to optimize management.

It seems that combination of experimental pain measures, clinical pain measures, serological biomarkers, and psychological features can be used for subgrouping patients into different sensitization classes.

Such a biomarker platform is adequate for diagnostic profiling purposes, predicting outcome after surgery and for profiling new analgesic compounds under development.

## REFERENCES


1. Ali A, Sundberg M, Robertsson O, Dahlberg LE, Thorstensson CA, Redlund-Johnell I, Kristiansson I, Lindstrand A. Dissatisfied patients after total knee arthroplasty. Acta Orthop 2014;85:229–33.
2. Arendt-Nielsen L. Central sensitization in humans: assessment and pharmacology. Handb Exp Pharmacol 2015;227:79–102.
3. Arendt-Nielsen L, Egsgaard LL, Petersen KK, Eskehave TN, Graven-Nielsen T, Hoeck HC, Simonsen O. A mechanism-based pain sensitivity index to characterize knee osteoarthritis patients with different disease stages and pain levels. Eur J Pain 2015;19:1406–17.
4. Arendt-Nielsen L, Eskehave TN, Egsgaard LL, Petersen KK, Graven-Nielsen T, Hoeck HC, Simonsen O, Siebuhr AS, Karsdal M, Bay-Jensen AC. Association between experimental pain biomarkers and serologic markers in patients with different degrees of painful knee osteoarthritis. Arthritis Rheumatol 2014;66:3317–26.
5. Arendt-Nielsen L, Graven-Nielsen T. Translational musculoskeletal pain research. Best Pract Res Clin Rheumatol 2011;25:209–26.
6. Arendt-Nielsen L, Hoeck HC. Optimizing the early phase development of new analgesics by human pain biomarkers. Expert Rev Neurother 2011;11:1631–51.
7. Arendt-Nielsen L, Nie H, Laursen MB, Laursen BS, Madeleine P, Simonsen OH, Graven-Nielsen T. Sensitization in patients with painful knee osteoarthritis. Pain 2010;149:573–81.
8. Arendt-Nielsen L, Nielsen TA, Gazerani P. Translational pain biomarkers in the early development of new neurotherapeutics for pain management. Expert Rev Neurother 2014;14:241–54.
9. Arendt-Nielsen L, Skou ST, Nielsen TA, Petersen KK. Altered central sensitization and pain modulation in the CNS in chronic joint pain. Curr Osteoporos Rep 2015;13:225–34.
10. Arendt-Nielsen L, Yarnitsky D. Experimental and clinical applications of quantitative sensory testing applied to skin, muscles and viscera. J Pain 2009;10:556–72.
11. Arrowsmith J. Phase II failures: 2008–2010. Nat Rev Drug Discov 2011;10:1.

12. Bartley EJ, King CD, Sibille KT, Cruz-Almeida Y, Riley JL III, Glover TL, Goodin BR, Sotolongo AS, Herbert MS, Bulls HW, et al. Enhanced pain sensitivity among individuals with symptomatic knee osteoarthritis: potential sex differences in central sensitization. Arthritis Care Res (Hoboken) 2016;68(4):472-80.
13. Bay-Jensen A, Liu Q, Byrjalsen I, Li Y, Wang J, Pedersen C, Leeming DJ, Dam EB, Zheng Q, Qvist P, Karsdal MA. Enzyme-linked immunosorbent assay (ELISAs) for metalloproteinase derived type II collagen neoepitope, CIIM: increased serum CIIM in subjects with severe radiographic osteoarthritis. Clin Biochem 2011;44:423–9.
14. Beswick AD, Wylde V, Gooberman-Hill R, Blom A, Dieppe P. What proportion of patients report long-term pain after total hip or knee replacement for osteoarthritis? A systematic review of prospective studies in unselected patients. BMJ Open 2012;2:e000435.
15. Binderup AT, Arendt-Nielsen L, Madeleine P. Pressure pain sensitivity maps of the neck-shoulder and the low back regions in men and women. BMC Musculoskelet Disord 2010;11:234.
16. Biurrun Manresa JA, Fritsche R, Vuilleumier PH, Oehler C, Mørch CD, Arendt-Nielsen L, Andersen OK, Curatolo M. Is the conditioned pain modulation paradigm reliable? A test–retest assessment using the nociceptive withdrawal reflex. PLoS One 2014;9:e100241.
17. Buvanendran A, Kroin JS, Della Valle CJ, Kari M, Moric M, Tuman KJ. Perioperative oral pregabalin reduces chronic pain after total knee arthroplasty: a prospective, randomized, controlled trial. Anesth Analg 2010;110:199–207.
18. Cruz-Almeida Y, King CD, Goodin BR, Sibille KT, Glover TL, Riley JL, Sotolongo A, Herbert MS, Schmidt J, Fessler BJ, et al. Psychological profiles and pain characteristics of older adults with knee osteoarthritis. Arthritis Care Res (Hoboken) 2013;65:1786–94.
19. Curatolo M, Arendt-Nielsen L. Central hypersensitivity in chronic musculoskeletal pain. Phys Med Rehabil Clin N Am 2015;26:175–84.
20. Dam EB, Byrjalsen I, Arendt-Nielsen L, Christiansen C, Karsdal MA. Relationships between knee pain and osteoarthritis biomarkers based on systemic fluids and magnetic resonance imaging. J Musculoskelet Pain 2011;19:144–53.
21. Davis MA, Ettinger WH, Neuhaus JM, Barclay JD, Segal MR. Correlates of knee pain among US adults with and without radiographic knee osteoarthritis. J Rheumatol 1992;19:1943–49.
22. Driban JB, Sitler MR, Barbe MF, Balasubramanian E. Is osteoarthritis a heterogeneous disease that can be stratified into subsets? Clin Rheumatol 2010;29:123–31.
23. Dye SF, Vaupel GL, Dye CC. Conscious neurosensory mapping of the internal structures of the human knee without intraarticular anesthesia. Am J Sports Med 1998;26:773–7.
24. Egsgaard LL, Eskehave TN, Bay-Jensen AC, Hoeck HC, Arendt-Nielsen L. Identifying specific profiles in patients with different degrees of painful knee osteoarthritis based on serological biochemical and mechanistic pain biomarkers: a diagnostic approach based on cluster analysis. Pain 2015;156:96–107.

25. Eitner A, Pester J, Nietzsche S, Hofmann GO, Schaible HG. The innervation of synovium of human osteoarthritic joints in comparison with normal rat and sheep synovium. Osteoarthritis Cartilage 2013;21:1383–91.
26. Eyre DR, Muir H. Type III collagen: a major constituent of rheumatoid and normal human synovial membrane. Connect Tissue Res 1975;4:11–16.
27. Farrell M, Gibson S, McMeeken J, Helme R. Pain and hyperalgesia in osteoarthritis of the hands. J Rheumatol 2000;27:441–7.
28. Fernández-de-las-Peñas C, Madeleine P, Cuadrado ML, Ge HY, Arendt-Nielsen L, Pareja JA. Pressure pain sensitivity mapping of the temporalis muscle revealed bilateral pressure hyperalgesia in patients with strictly unilateral migraine. Cephalalgia 2009;29:670–6.
29. Finan PH, Buenaver LF, Bounds SC, Hussain S, Park RJ, Haque UJ, Campbell CM, Haythornthwaite JA, Edwards RR, Smith MT. Discordance between pain and radiographic severity in knee osteoarthritis: findings from quantitative sensory testing of central sensitization. Arthritis Rheum 2013;65:363–72.
30. Fingleton C, Smart K, Moloney N, Fullen BM, Doody C. Pain sensitization in people with knee osteoarthritis: a systematic review and meta-analysis. Osteoarthritis Cartilage 2015;23:1043–56.
31. Gandhi R, Santone D, Takahashi M, Dessouki O, Mahomed NN. Inflammatory predictors of ongoing pain 2 years following knee replacement surgery. Knee 2013;20:316–8.
32. Grässel SG. The role of peripheral nerve fibers and their neurotransmitters in cartilage and bone physiology and pathophysiology. Arthritis Res Ther 2014; 16:485.
33. Graven-Nielsen T, Vaegter HB, Finocchietti S, Handberg G, Arendt-Nielsen L. Assessment of musculoskeletal pain sensitivity and temporal summation by cuff pressure algometry: a reliability study. Pain 2015;156:2193–202.
34. Graven-Nielsen T, Wodehouse T, Langford RM, Arendt-Nielsen L, Kidd BL. Normalization of widespread hyperesthesia and facilitated spatial summation of deep-tissue pain in knee osteoarthritis patients after knee replacement. Arthritis Rheum 2012;64:2907–16.
35. Gwilym SE, Keltner JR, Warnaby CE, Carr AJ, Chizh B, Chessell I, Tracey I. Psychophysical and functional imaging evidence supporting the presence of central sensitization in a cohort of osteoarthritis patients. Arthritis Rheum 2009;61:1226–34.
36. Hannan MT, Felson DT, Pincus T. Analysis of the discordance between radiographic changes and knee pain in osteoarthritis of the knee. J Rheumatol 2000;27:1513–17.
37. Harden RN, Wallach G, Gagnon CM, Zereshki A, Mukai A, Saracoglu M, Kuroda MM, Graciosa JR, Bruehl S. The osteoarthritis knee model: psychophysical characteristics and putative outcomes. J Pain 2013;14:281–9.
38. Hendiani JA, Westlund KN, Lawand N, Goel N, Lisse J, McNearney T. Mechanical sensation and pain thresholds in patients with chronic arthropathies. J Pain 2003;4:203–11.

39. Hinman RS, Crossley KM. Patellofemoral joint osteoarthritis: an important subgroup of knee osteoarthritis. Rheumatology (Oxford) 2007;46:1057–62.
40. Imamura M, Ezquerro F, Marcon Alfieri F, Vilas Boas L, Tozetto-Mendoza TR, Chen J, Özçakar L, Arendt-Nielsen L, Rizzo Battistella L. Serum levels of proinflammatory cytokines in painful knee osteoarthritis and sensitization. Int J Inflam 2015;2015:329792.
41. Imamura M, Imamura ST, Kaziyama HH, Targino RA, Hsing WT, de Souza LP, Cutait MM, Fregni F, Camanho GL. Impact of nervous system hyperalgesia on pain, disability, and quality of life in patients with knee osteoarthritis: a controlled analysis. Arthritis Rheum 2008;59:1424–31.
42. Ishijima M, Watari T, Naito K, Kaneko H, Futami I, Yoshimura-Ishida K, Tomonaga A, Yamaguchi H, Yamamoto T, Nagaoka I, et al. Relationships between biomarkers of cartilage, bone, synovial metabolism and knee pain provide insights into the origins of pain in early knee osteoarthritis. Arthritis Res Ther 2011;13:R22.
43. Jensen K, Andersen HØ, Olesen J, Lindblom U. Pressure-pain threshold in human temporal region. Evaluation of a new pressure algometer. Pain 1986;25:313–23.
44. Jespersen A, Dreyer L, Kendall S, Graven-Nielsen T, Arendt-Nielsen L, Bliddal H, Danneskiold-Samsoe B. Computerized cuff pressure algometry: a new method to assess deep-tissue hypersensitivity in fibromyalgia. Pain 2007;131:57–62.
45. Kehlet H, Jensen TS, Woolf CJ. Persistent postsurgical pain: risk factors and prevention. Lancet 2006;367:1618–25.
46. King CD, Sibille KT, Goodin BR, Cruz-Almeida Y, Glover TL, Bartley E, Riley JL, Herbert MS, Sotolongo A, Schmidt J, et al. Experimental pain sensitivity differs as a function of clinical pain severity in symptomatic knee osteoarthritis. Osteoarthritis Cartilage 2013;21:1243–52.
47. Kissin I. The development of new analgesics over the past 50 years: a lack of real breakthrough drugs. Anesth Analg 2010;110:780–9.
48. Knoop J, van der Leeden M, Thorstensson CA, Roorda LD, Lems WF, Knol DL, Steultjens MP, Dekker J. Identification of phenotypes with different clinical outcomes in knee osteoarthritis: data from the Osteoarthritis Initiative. Arthritis Care Res 2011;63:1535–42.
49. Kosek E, Ordeberg G. Lack of pressure pain modulation by heterotopic noxious conditioning stimulation in patients with painful osteoarthritis before, but not following, surgical pain relief. Pain 2000;88:69–78.
50. Kosek E, Roos EM, Ageberg E, Nilsdotter A. Increased pain sensitivity but normal function of exercise induced analgesia in hip and knee osteoarthritis: treatment effects of neuromuscular exercise and total joint replacement. Osteoarthritis Cartilage 2013;21:1299–307.
51. Kuni B, Wang H, Rickert M, Ewerbeck V, Schiltenwolf M. Pain threshold correlates with functional scores in osteoarthritis patients. Acta Orthop 2015;86:215–9.
52. Kurtz S, Ong K, Lau E, Mowat F, Halpern M. Projections of primary and revision hip and knee arthroplasty in the United States from 2005 to 2030. J Bone Joint Surg Am 2007;89:780–5.

53. Kushner I. C-reactive protein and the acute-phase response. Hosp Pract (Off Ed). 1990;25:13, 16, 21–8.
54. Larmer PJ, Reay ND, Aubert ER, Kersten P. Systematic review of guidelines for the physical management of osteoarthritis. Arch Phys Med Rehabil 2014;95:375–89.
55. Lee YC, Lu B, Bathon JM, Haythornthwaite JA, Smith MT, Page GG, Edwards RR. Pain sensitivity and pain reactivity in osteoarthritis. Arthritis Care Res (Hoboken) 2011;63:320–7.
56. Lewis GN, Rice DA, McNair PJ. Conditioned pain modulation in populations with chronic pain: a systematic review and meta-analysis. J Pain 2012;13:936–44.
57. Lluch E, Torres R, Nijs J, Van OJ. Evidence for central sensitization in patients with osteoarthritis pain: a systematic literature review. Eur J Pain 2014;18:1367–75.
58. Lovell C, Nicholls A, Jayson M, Bailey A. Changes in the collagen of synovial membrane in rheumatoid arthritis and effect of D-penicillamine. Clin Sci 1978;55:31–40.
59. Lundblad H, Kreicbergs A, Jansson KA. Prediction of persistent pain after total knee replacement for osteoarthritis. J Bone Joint Surg Br 2008;90:166–71.
60. Macrae WA. Chronic post-surgical pain: 10 years on. Br J Anaesth 2008;101:77–86.
61. Morgan P, Van Der Graaf PH, Arrowsmith J, Feltner DE, Drummond KS, Wegner CD, Street SD. Can the flow of medicines be improved? Fundamental pharmacokinetic and pharmacological principles toward improving Phase II survival. Drug Discov Today 2012;17:419–24.
62. Mutlu EK, Ozdincler AR. Reliability and responsiveness of algometry for measuring pressure pain threshold in patients with knee osteoarthritis. J Phys Ther Sci 2015;27:1961–5.
63. Neogi T, Felson D, Niu J, Nevitt M, Lewis CE, Aliabadi P, Sack B, Torner J, Bradley L, Zhang Y. Association between radiographic features of knee osteoarthritis and pain: results from two cohort studies. BMJ 2009;339:b2844.
64. Neogi T, Frey-Law L, Scholz J, Niu J, Arendt-Nielsen L, Woolf C, Nevitt M, Bradley L, Felson DT; Multicenter Osteoarthritis (MOST) Study. Sensitivity and sensitisation in relation to pain severity in knee osteoarthritis: trait or state? Ann Rheum Dis 2015;74:682–8.
65. Nie H, Arendt-Nielsen L, Andersen H, Graven-Nielsen T. Temporal summation of pain evoked by mechanical stimulation in deep and superficial tissue. J Pain 2005;6:348–55.
66. Oono Y, Nie H, Matos RVL, Wang K, Arendt-Nielsen L. The inter- and intra-individual variance in descending pain modulation evoked by different conditioning stimuli in healthy men. Scand J Pain 2011;2:162–9.
67. Osgood E, Trudeau JJ, Eaton TA, Jensen MP, Gammaitoni A, Simon LS, Katz N. Development of a bedside pain assessment kit for the classification of patients with osteoarthritis. Rheumatol Int 2015;35:1005–13.
68. Pearle AD, Scanzello CR, George S, Mandl LA, DiCarlo EF, Peterson M, Peterson M, Sculco TP, Crow MK. Elevated high-sensitivity C-reactive protein levels are associated with local inflammatory findings in patients with osteoarthritis. Osteoarthritis Cartilage 2007;15:516–23.

69. Pelletier JP, Martel-Pelletier J, Abramson SB. Osteoarthritis, an inflammatory disease: potential implication for the selection of new therapeutic targets. Arthritis Rheum 2001;44:1237–47.
70. Petersen KK, Arendt-Nielsen L, Simonsen O, Wilder-Smith O, Laursen MB. Presurgical assessment of temporal summation of pain predicts the development of chronic postoperative pain 12 months after total knee replacement. Pain 2015;156:55–61.
71. Petersen KK, Simonsen O, Laursen MB, Nielsen TA, Rasmussen S, Arendt-Nielsen L. Chronic postoperative pain after primary and revision total knee arthroplasty. Clin J Pain 2015;31:1–6.
72. Rakel B, Vance C, Zimmerman MB, Petsas-Blodgett N, Amendola A, Sluka KA. Mechanical hyperalgesia and reduced quality of life occur in people with mild knee osteoarthritis pain. Clin J Pain 2015;31:315–22.
73. Rutjes AW, Jüni P, da Costa BR, Trelle S, Nüesch E, Reichenbach S. Viscosupplementation for osteoarthritis of the knee: a systematic review and meta-analysis. Ann Intern Med 2012;157:180–91.
74. Siebuhr AS, Petersen KK, Arendt-Nielsen L, Egsgaard LL, Eskehave T, Christiansen C, Simonsen O, Hoeck HC, Karsdal MA, Bay-Jensen AC. Identification and characterisation of osteoarthritis patients with inflammation derived tissue turnover. Osteoarthritis Cartilage 2014;22:44–50.
75. Skjøt-Arkil H, Schett G, Zhang C, Larsen DV, Wang Y, Zheng Q, Larsen MR, Nawrocki A, Bay-Jensen AC, Henriksen K, et al. Investigation of two novel biochemical markers of inflammation, matrix metalloproteinase and cathepsin generated fragments of C-reactive protein, in patients with ankylosing spondylitis. Clin Exp Rheumatol 2012;30:371–9.
76. Skou ST, Graven-Nielsen T, Lengsoe L, Simonsen O, Laursen MB, Arendt-Nielsen L. Relating clinical measures of pain with experimentally assessed pain mechanisms in patients with knee osteoarthritis. Scand J Pain 2013;4:111–7.
77. Skou ST, Graven-Nielsen T, Rasmussen S, Simonsen OH, Laursen MB, Arendt-Nielsen L. Widespread sensitization in patients with chronic pain after revision total knee arthroplasty. Pain 2013;154:1588–94.
78. Skou ST, Graven-Nielsen T, Rasmussen S, Simonsen OH, Laursen MB, Arendt-Nielsen L. Facilitation of pain sensitization in knee osteoarthritis and persistent post-operative pain: a cross-sectional study. Eur J Pain 2014;18:1024–31.
79. Skou ST, Thomsen H, Simonsen OH. The value of routine radiography in patients with knee osteoarthritis consulting primary health care: a study of agreement. Eur J Gen Pract 2014;20:10–16.
80. Suokas AK, Walsh DA, McWilliams DF, Condon L, Moreton B, Wylde V, Arendt-Nielsen L, Zhang W. Quantitative sensory testing in painful osteoarthritis: a systematic review and meta-analysis. Osteoarthritis Cartilage 2012;20:1075–85.
81. Uthman OA, van der Windt DA, Jordan JL, Dziedzic KS, Healey EL, Peat GM, Foster NE. Exercise for lower limb osteoarthritis: systematic review incorporating trial sequential analysis and network meta-analysis. BMJ 2013;347:f5555.
82. van der Esch M, Knoop J, van der Leeden M, Roorda LD, Lems WF, Knol DL, Dekker J. Clinical phenotypes in patients with knee osteoarthritis: a study in the Amsterdam osteoarthritis cohort. Osteoarthritis Cartilage 2015;23:544–9.

83. Wandel S, Jüni P, Tendal B, Nüesch E, Villiger PM, Welton NJ, Reichenbach S, Trelle S. Effects of glucosamine, chondroitin, or placebo in patients with osteoarthritis of hip or knee: network meta-analysis. BMJ 2010;341:c4675.
84. Wenham CY, Conaghan PG. The role of synovitis in osteoarthritis. Ther Adv Musculoskelet Dis 2010;2:349–59.
85. Wessel J. The reliability and validity of pain threshold measurements in osteoarthritis of the knee. Scand J Rheumatol 1995;24:238–42.
86. Wylde V, Palmer S, Learmonth ID, Dieppe P. Somatosensory abnormalities in knee OA. Rheumatology (Oxford) 2012;51:535–43.
87. Wylde V, Palmer S, Learmonth ID, Dieppe P. Test-retest reliability of Quantitative Sensory Testing in knee osteoarthritis and healthy participants. Osteoarthritis Cartilage 2011;19:655–8.
88. Wylde V, Palmer S, Learmonth ID, Dieppe P. The association between pre-operative pain sensitisation and chronic pain after knee replacement: an exploratory study. Osteoarthritis Cartilage 2013;21:1253–6.
89. Wylde V, Sayers A, Lenguerrand E, Gooberman-Hill R, Pyke M, Beswick AD, Dieppe P, Blom AW. Preoperative widespread pain sensitization and chronic pain after hip and knee replacement: a cohort analysis. Pain 2015;156:47–54.

CHAPTER 9

# Osteoarthritis Pain: From Pathophysiology to Clinical Characteristics

*Serge Perrot*

In Europe, 20% of chronic pain is related to osteoarthritis (OA) [45], and pain is the main symptom in OA. Furthermore, pain related to OA is considered as the prototypical chronic nociceptive pain condition, and used as one major clinical model for the development of new analgesics dedicated to chronic pain.

In 420 BC, Hippocrates described the Rheuma theory: Joint pain is driven by the brain. It describes that when brain sends more liquid to the lower parts of the body that induces pain in the hip to finally reach all the joints [23]. This theory is now being revisited in the 21st century with neurosciences, describing all influences of neurologic system in joint disorders.

Pain is a ubiquitous symptom in osteoarticular diseases [27], especially in OA [6], much more prevalent than stiffness and disability. OA frequency is increasing, mostly related to age and obesity. Paradoxically, compared with inflammation and immunity research, for many years, joint pain pathophysiology has not been extensively studied. OA pain has been considered as a prototypical nociceptive pain condition, and clinicians have expected that pain can be an alarm signal, correlated with the intensity of joint degradation [14]. In OA, most authors have focused their studies more on joint architecture and local degradation than on pain, but we will see that it may have neuropathic component, and it is not a stable and continuous symptom [47].

OA pain pathophysiology is a recent subject for researchers, and as in other clinical pain conditions, we will see that OA pain pathophysiology includes four different processes:

- Transduction: conversion of energy induced by a painful stimulus (mechanical, thermal, chemical) into electrical energy by specific receptors
- Transmission: from periphery to centers (spinal cord and brain), with specific pathways
- Perception in the brain cortical zones
- Modulation by brain and spinal structures, by inhibiting and facilitating ways. This phenomenon is crucial not only to reduce pain sensation, but also to develop chronicity.

We will see that OA pain is a complex phenomenon, involving peripheral and central mechanisms, modulated by many factors, including psychological [18] and genetic factors [56]. Recent findings of neuroimaging have improved knowledge in these mechanisms, and new treatments may be proposed in the next future for better management.

## EXPERIMENTAL PAIN MODELS: IS THERE A MODEL OF OA PAIN?

In OA pain, as in any pain conditions, research on animal models has tried to be as close as possible to the human condition. In fact, experimental studies on OA pain have been mostly developed in inflammatory models, especially in arthritis, comparing data in arthritic and control animals. Parallel to OA pain, several models of OA have been described, but these models have been initially developed to analyze structural joint changes rather than to analyze nociceptive sensations in animals. Recently, few models have also been developed to analyze nociceptive pain behavior, after cruciate ligament transection, meniscectomy, and monoiodoacetate injection [39, 62]. However, the most frequent animal models of chronic joint pain are inflammatory models like the models of Freund's adjuvant injection [7], carrageenan plantar injection [35], or urate joint injection [15].

Experimental tests that can assess nociceptive behavior in animals are mostly represented by mechanical stimuli, like the Randall and Selitto test [49], or thermal stimuli, like immerging hind paw in different temperatures. Other tests are based on observations of spontaneous behavior: motility, writhing. . . As in all animal studies, translation to human being is limited, and many animal findings have not been confirmed in human [8].

## NEUROANATOMY OF JOINT AND PERIPHERAL MECHANISMS OF OA PAIN

Origin of joint pain has been unknown for a long period of time. In 1945, Davies reported the first experimental joint pain and noted that synovium was insensitive to pressure but that needles puncture induced diffuse intra-articular pain [16]. In 1950, Kellgren and Samuel [34] studied pain induced by needles in the knee of healthy volunteers; they demonstrated that synovium was insensitive to needles punctures but that capsule and ligaments were sensitive to pain.

Immunostaining has demonstrated the type of innervation of the joint [38]. Capsule, ligaments, meniscus, periosteum, and subchondral bone are largely innervated by a dense network of myelinic and amyelinic fibers. Synovium is mostly innervated by amyelinic fibers, although cartilage has no innervation [22].

In the joint, there are four types of sensory organs [38]. Type I and II receptors, that are corpuscular organs (Paccini, Golgi, Ruffini), are localized in the capsule, ligaments, and meniscus, but not in the synovium. There are mechanoreceptors, sensitive to pressure and traction, transmitting the message by myelinic fibers. Type III receptors, formed by thin Aδ myelinic fibers, are located on ligament surface and act as mechanoreceptors of high threshold, answering to strong mechanical stimuli and to a lower degree to thermal stimuli.

Type IV receptors, also called polymodals, are formed by free terminals of unmyelinated C fibers and are representing the most important type of joint receptors in all structures but absent in the cartilage. They are normally not activated and are called polymodals because they are activated by mechanical, thermal, and chemical stimuli in pathological conditions such as inflammation. Type III and IV receptors are involved in pain sensation induced by joint lesions. They are also sensitized by increased intra-articular pressure and by chemical local changes.

## TRANSDUCTION: PERIPHERAL STIMULI AND RECEPTORS IN OA PAIN

More than 80% of the fibers in the joint are unmyelinated fibers, equally distributed between C fibers and sympathetic fibers [9, 38].

### Mechanical Stimuli Induce Joint Pain

One important component of OA pain is mechanical pain. In a normal joint, intra-articular pressure is between 2 and 10 mm Hg [37]. In case of inflammation or local articular lesion, pressure can increase up to 20 mm Hg. Cartilage damage may induce hyperpressure of subchondral bone [55]. In the joint, there are specific nociceptors that are specifically activated by mechanical stimulus [29].

### Inflammatory Stimuli Induce OA Pain

In the joint, even in OA, local inflammation with release of phospholipases, cyclooxygenases, lipoxygenases, leukotrienes, free radicals, and NO [33] is involved in pain mechanisms.

### Joint Receptors and Pain Mediators

In the joint, C fibers, also called peptidergic, express the TrkA receptor for NGF (neuronal growth factor), P2X3 receptor for adenosine triphosphate, and also GDNF (glial-derived neurotrophic factor) receptor. Mediators of these fibers are substance P, calcitonin gene-related peptide (CGRP), neuropeptide Y (NPY) [1], and VIP [41] in all joint structures except the cartilage. NGF is an important component of the C fibers, with an important role in joint pain [3, 57], currently targeted by new biological therapies [28].

Recently, receptors that play a role in neuropathic pain have also been found in the joint: TRPV receptors are present in many joint structures and can be the target of descending inhibitory mechanisms [13].

Aside nociceptors, other receptors in the joint may take part in the mechanisms of joint pain, and can represent putative targets for analgesic therapies: Opioid receptors present in the joint [43], as cannabinoid receptors [36], increased with inflammation. This has suggested the possible use of local morphine in joint pain [53].

## TRANSMISSION OF PAIN: FROM PERIPHERY TO THE BRAIN

Pain has a complex pathophysiology, and in OA, recent findings have demonstrated the important role of central mechanisms. In OA, there is increasing evidence that central mechanisms play a role in pain sensation. When injecting a saline solution in anterior tibialis muscle, patients with knee OA experience more intense and more diffuse pain compared with normal controls [4].

In fact, there are probably both peripheral and central mechanisms at different stages: peripheral mechanisms more in the early stage and central mechanisms more in late and chronic stages [2]. Interactions between central and peripheral system suggest a general plasticity of nociceptive system in OA pain [21, 30]. This plasticity may depend on different factors (e.g., emotional factors).

### Brain Activation in OA Pain

Recent findings have demonstrated that different types of pain could be related to some activation in different brain regions: Spontaneous pain could be mainly related to medial prefrontal–limbic cortical areas, which are regions involved in emotional status. Conversely, stimulus-evoked pain could be more related to somatosensory nociceptive processing regions [46].

### Brain Sensitization and Modifications

Recent findings in OA pain have demonstrated brain activation and brain volume modifications in patients with chronic pain related to OA. Some studies have analyzed brain activation and have demonstrated that OA pain, as most chronic pain states, is associated with central sensitization. Clinically, central sensitization related to joint pain induces pain for stimuli that currently do not induce pain (allodynia), with larger area of pain activation and longer duration of pain [2]. Central sensitization in OA has been confirmed by quantitative sensory testing (QST) analyses and functional MRI [24]. More recent studies have analyzed brain volume, specifically in some areas, and found some modifications in the gray matter: As in other chronic pain states, OA is associated with decrease of gray matter [50, 52], but this decrease may not be permanent because gray matter is regenerated 6–9 months after effective hip or knee surgery [24, 50].

## PERCEPTION OF OA PAIN AND CORRELATION WITH JOINT DAMAGE

One constant question in OA, both for patients and physicians, is related to the correlation between pain and joint damage. Many patients and their physicians believe that pain is correlated with joint damage and that intense pain may reflect a high degree of joint degeneration.

Cohort studies have demonstrated that there is a poor correlation between pain intensity in OA and the degree of joint degeneration. In a study pooling two cohorts, the MOST and the Framingham cohort, Neogi et al. [44] have demonstrated that pain was more correlated with joint-space narrowing than with the presence of osteophytes. They also found that only high degrees of joint deterioration were associated with higher pain levels. A more precise study has analyzed all joint components by MRI study to investigate which structural changes were mostly associated with pain in OA [59]; the authors demonstrated that synovitis and bone marrow edema were the structural changes that were most correlated with pain, whereas osteophytes, bone cysts, meniscal changes, and ligament tears were not associated with OA pain. In conclusion to this question, one may answer that on an individual basis, it is still not relevant to correlate pain with joint damage.

## CLINICAL EXPRESSION OF OA PAIN

Very few papers have described pain dimensions in OA, with little consensus on its dimensions [5]. Pain intensity in OA is currently assessed by numerical and visual analog scale, to assess its intensity [25]. The MacGill Pain Questionnaire (MPQ) has two different subscales—sensorial and emotional—that may be used to differentiate both components, and has been validated in patients with hip and knee OA [19].

Some authors have analyzed night pain in knee OA [60] and patient's views on knee OA pain [31]. A recent initiative from Osteoarthritis Research Society International and OMERACT (Outcome Measures in Rheumatology) has investigated several dimensions in OA pain, providing ICOAP (Intermittent and Constant OsteoArthritis Pain), a new questionnaire including pain intensity, frequency, and impact on mood, sleep, and quality of life [26]. This qualitative approach explored changes in pain characteristics over time, in relation with priorities and concerns of individuals living with hip or knee pain. Authors of this study have defined two distinct pain conditions in OA, related to the context of OA progression, with intermittent and intense pain having the greatest impact on quality of life. Although several pain descriptors are proposed in this chapter, these descriptors were not intended to be specifically used to define pain phenotypes in OA as it has been done in neuropathic pain. In this line, we have developed a qualitative analysis of OA pain with a new questionnaire, the OsteoArthritis Symptom Inventory Scale (OASIS), to characterize pain quality in OA and, in the future, to help define different phenotypes of OA pain [11].

## NEUROPATHIC CHARACTERISTICS AND SENSITIZATION IN OA PAIN

Recently, neuropathic characteristics have been investigated in painful OA, with different questionnaires such as PainDETECT and Leeds Assessment of Neuropathic Signs and Symptoms. Most studies have concluded that neuropathic component is found in around one-third of the patients with painful OA [17], and some have also found that it could be associated with augmented central pain processing [42]. These neuropathic characteristics are associated with higher intensity scores and are a significant contributor to decreased quality of life. Other authors have found that neuropathic characteristics were associated with meniscal lesions [51]. The question of OA pain as a neuropathic pain in some patients has been raised based on these studies. In fact, neuropathic pain is classified as pain caused by a lesion or disease of the somatosensory nervous system. Neuropathy could contribute directly to OA knee pain through peripheral nerve damage within the joint, but there is currently no test by which to identify neuropathy within articular nociceptive pathways. In one cross-sectional study on OA pain characteristics, authors have found an association with previous history of knee surgery and neuropathic symptoms, suggesting that some of the NP-like symptoms may result from nerve damage. Although several symptoms may suggest neuropathic mechanisms, it remains uncertain which questionnaire or which cutoff is most accurate in identifying neuropathic pain mechanisms in OA. In all cases, central processing observed in OA pain may augment pain severity and contribute to overlapping pain qualities associated with either nerve damage or joint damage.

Pain assessment has recently integrated more comprehensive measurements, like QST. In OA, several studies have analyzed pain thresholds and pain sensitivity to different stimuli [54], and have confirmed the role of central sensitization [61].

## FACTORS THAT INFLUENCE OA PAIN

One major OA pain specificity is the influence of exercise and movement on OA pain. Movement may increase pain, but exercise is a major nonpharmacological approach of OA pain. Thus, exercise type and dose are very important to consider [32].

Pain is a subjective experience, with different strategies to cope with OA pain [48], regarding the site of OA pain. OA pain, more than other pain conditions, is a condition in which lots of influences have been reported by patients. Weather conditions may influence OA pain sensitivity, with differences according to age, gender, and countries [58].

Hormonal changes may also represent factors that increase the severity of pain [10], as seen in the menopausal age. Vitamin D deficiency has been considered as a putative factor for OA pain flares but not confirmed in prospective studies [40]. Genetic factors may also modify pain, and also morphine consumption required for analgesic purpose in knee OA [12].

Lastly, OA pain is a condition in which mutual influences between pain and mood disturbances should be analyzed in patients' management [20].

## CONCLUSIONS

Pain in OA has a complex pathophysiology, related but distinct from OA pathophysiology. In this pathophysiology, the joint is as important as the brain and as all modulating systems. It is recent that pain physicians and rheumatologists are sharing their research to better understand this major symptom in OA. This has led to the better description of multiple mechanisms. All mechanisms are important to consider when treating OA, for a better management of the patients, and may be taken into account in the research of specific analgesic treatments.

## DISCLOSURE

The author has received consultant fees from Pfizer, Lilly, Grunenthal, Astellas, Sanofi, BMS, and Roche in the last 5 years.

## REFERENCES


1. Ahmed M, Bjurholm A, Schultzberg M, Theodorsson E, Kreicbergs A. Increased levels of substance P and calcitonin gene-related peptide in rat adjuvant arthritis: a combined immunohistochemical and radioimmunoassay analysis. Arthritis Rheum 1995;38:699–709.
2. Arendt-Nielsen L, Nie H, Laursen MB, Laursen BS, Madeleine P, Simonsen OH, Graven-Nielsen T. Sensitization in patients with painful knee osteoarthritis. Pain 2010;149:573–81.
3. Ashraf S, Mapp PI, Burston J, Bennett AJ, Chapman V, Walsh DA. Augmented pain behavioural responses to intra-articular injection of nerve growth factor in two animal models of osteoarthritis. Ann Rheum Dis 2013;73:1710–8. doi:10.1136/annrheumdis-2013-203416.
4. Bajaj P, Bajaj P, Graven-Nielsen T, Arendt-Nielsen L. Osteoarthritis and its association with muscle hyperalgesia: an experimental controlled study. Pain 2001;93:107–14.
5. Bellamy N, Sothern RB, Campbell J. Rhythmic variations in pain perception in osteoarthritis of the knee. J Rheumatol 1990;17:364–72.
6. Burckhardt C. The use of the McGill Pain Questionnaire in assessing arthritis pain. Pain 1984;19:305–14.
7. Calvino B, Crepon-Bernard MO, Le Bars D. Parallel clinical and behavioural studies of adjuvant-induced arthritis in the rat: possible relationship with "chronic pain." Behav Brain Res 1987;24:11–29.
8. Casey KL, Dubner R. Animal models of chronic pain, scientific and ethical issues. Pain 1989;38:249–52.
9. Catre MG, Salo PT. Quantitative analysis of the sympathetic innervation of the rat knee joint. J Anat 1999;194:233–9.
10. Cauley JA, Kwoh CK, Egeland G, Nevitt MC, Cooperstein L, Rohay J, Towers A, Gutai JP. Serum sex hormones and severity of osteoarthritis of the hand. J Rheumatol 1993;20:1170–5.
11. Cedraschi C, Delézay S, Marty M, Berenbaum F, Bouhassira D, Henrotin Y, Laroche F, Perrot S. "Let's talk about OA pain": a qualitative analysis of the perceptions of people suffering from OA. Towards the development of a specific pain OA-related questionnaire, the Osteoarthritis Symptom Inventory Scale (OASIS). PLoS One 2013;8:e79988.
12. Chou W, Yang L, Lu H. Association of mu-opioid receptor gene polymorphism (A118G) with variations in morphine consumption for analgesia after total knee arthroplasty. Acta Anaesthesiol Scand 2006;50:787–92.
13. Chu KL, Chandran P, Joshi SK, Jarvis MF, Kym PR, McGaraughty S. TRPV1-related modulation of spinal neuronal activity and behavior in a rat model of osteoarthritic pain. Brain Res 2011;1369:158–66.
14. Claessens AAMC, Schouten JSAG, Van den Ouweland FA, Valkenburg HA. Do clinical findings associate with radiographic osteoarthritis of the knee? Ann Rheum Dis 1990;49:771–4.

15. Coderre TJ, Wall PD. Ankle joint urate arthritis (AJUA) in rats. An alternative animal model of arthritis to that proposed by Freund's adjuvant. Pain 1987:379–93.
16. Davies DV. Anatomy and physiology of diarthrodial joints. Ann Rheum Dis 1945;5:29–35.
17. Dimitroulas T, Duarte RV, Behura A, Kitas GD, Raphael JH. Neuropathic pain in osteoarthritis: a review of pathophysiological mechanisms and implications for treatment. Semin Arthritis Rheum 2014;44:145–54.
18. Edwards RR, Bingham CO III, Bathon J, Haythornthwaite JA. Catastrophizing and pain in arthritis, fibromyalgia, and other rheumatic diseases. Arthritis Rheum 2006;55:325–32.
19. Gandhi R, Tsvetkov D, Dhottar H, Davey JR, Mahomed NN. Quantifying the pain experience in hip and knee osteoarthritis. Pain Res Manag 2010;15: 224–8.
20. Goldenberg D. The interface of pain and mood disturbances in the rheumatic diseases. Semin Arthritis Rheum 2012;40:15–31.
21. Graven Nielsen T, Arendt Nielsen L. Peripheral and central sensitisation in musculoskeletal pain disorders: an experimental approach. Curr Rheumatol Rep 2002;4:313–21.
22. Grigg P. Properties of sensory neurons innervating synovial joints. Cells Tissues Organs 2001;169:218–25.
23. Grossman BJ. Rheumatoid arthritis from prehistory to Hippocrates. Proc Inst Med Chic 1966;26:114–5.
24. Gwilym SE, Keltner JR, Warnaby CE, Carr AJ, Chizh B, Chessell I, Tracey I. Psychophysical and functional imaging evidence supporting the presence of central sensitization in a cohort of osteoarthritis patients. Arthritis Rheum 2009;61:1226–34.
25. Hawker G, Mian S, Kendzerska T. Measures of adult pain. Arthritis Care Res 2011;63:S240–52.
26. Hawker GA, Davis AM, French MR, Cibere J, Jordan JM, March L, Suarez-Almazor M, Katz JN, Dieppe P. Development and preliminary psychometric testing of a new OA pain measure: an OARSI/OMERACT initiative. Osteoarthritis Cartilage 2008;16:409–14.
27. Hawley DJ, Wolfe F. Pain, disability and pain/disability relationships in seven rheumatic disorders: a study of 1,522 patients. J Rheumatol 1991;18:1552–7.
28. Hefti FF, Rosenthal A, Walicka PA, Wyatt S, Vergara G, Shelton DL, Davis AM. Novel class of pain drug based on antagonism of NGF. Trends Pharmacol Sci 2005;27:85–91.
29. Heppelmann B, McDougall JJ. Inhibitory effect of amiloride and gadolinium on fine afferent nerves in the rat knee: evidence of mechanogated ion channels in joints. Exp Brain Res 2005;167:114–8.
30. Imamura M, Imamura ST, Kaziyama HH, Targino RA, Hsing WT, de Souza LP, Cutait MM, Fregni F, Camanho GL. Impact of nervous system hyperalgesia on pain, disability, and quality of life in patients with knee osteoarthritis: a controlled analysis. Arthritis Rheum 2008;59:1424–31.

31. Jinks C, Ong BN, O'Neill T. "Well, it's nobody's responsibility but my own." A qualitative study to explore views about the determinants of health and prevention of knee pain in older adults. BMC Public Health 2010;10:148.
32. Juhl C, Christensen R, Roos EM, Zhang W, Lund H. Impact of exercise type and dose on pain and disability in knee osteoarthritis: a systematic review and meta-regression analysis of randomized controlled trials. Arthritis Rheumatol 2014;66:622–36.
33. Karsdal MA, Woodworth T, Henriksen K, Maksymowych WP, Genant H, Vergnaud P, Christiansen C, Schubert T, Qvist P, Schett G, et al. Biochemical markers of ongoing joint damage in rheumatoid arthritis—current and future applications, limitations and opportunities. Arthritis Res Ther 2011;13:215.
34. Kellgren JH, Samuel EP. The sensitivity and innervation of the articular capsule. J Bone Joint Surg (Br) 1950;32:84–92.
35. Lam FY, Ferrel WR. Inhibition of carageenan induced inflammation in the rat knee joint by substance P antagonist. Ann Rheum Dis 1989;48:928–32.
36. La Porta C, Bura SA, Aracil-Fernández A, Manzanares J, Maldonado R. Role of CB1 and CB2 cannabinoid receptors in the development of joint pain induced by monosodium iodoacetate. Pain 2013;154:160–74.
37. Levick JR. An investigation into the validity of subatmospheric pressure recordings from synovial fluid and their dependence on joint angle. J Physiol 1979;289:55–67.
38. Mapp PI. Innervation of the synovium. Ann Rheum Dis 1995;54:398–403.
39. Mapp PI, Sagar DR, Ashraf S, Burston JJ, Suri S, Chapman V, Walsh DA. Differences in structural and pain phenotypes in the sodium monoiodoacetate and meniscal transection models of osteoarthritis. Osteoarthritis Cartilage 2013;21:1336–45.
40. McAlindon T, LaValley M, Schneider E, Nuite M, Lee JY, Price LL, Lo G, Dawson-Hughes B. Effect of vitamine D supplementation on progression of knee pain and cartilage volume loss in patients with symptomatic osteoarthritis: a randomized controlled trial. JAMA 2013;9:155–62.
41. McDougall JJ, Watkins L, Li Z. Vasoactive intestinal peptide (VIP) is a modulator of joint pain in a rat model of osteoarthritis. Pain 2006;123:98–105.
42. Moreton BJ, Tew V, das Nair R, Wheeler M, Walsh DA, Lincoln NB. Pain phenotype in patients with knee osteoarthritis: classification and measurement properties of painDETECT and self-report Leeds assessment of neuropathic symptoms and signs scale in a cross-sectional study. Arthritis Care Res (Hoboken) 2015;67:519–28.
43. Mousa SA, Straub RH, Schäfer M, Stein C. Beta-endorphin, Met-enkephalin and corresponding opioid receptors within synovium of patients with joint trauma, osteoarthritis and rheumatoid arthritis. Ann Rheum Dis 2007;66:871–9.
44. Neogi T, Felson D, Niu J, Nevitt M, Lewis CE, Aliabadi P, Sack B, Torner J, Bradley L, Zhang Y. Association between radiographic features of knee osteoarthritis and pain: results from two cohort studies. BMJ 2009;339:b2844.
45. O'Brien T, Breivik H. The impact of chronic pain: European patient's perspective over 12 months. Scand J Pain 2012;3:23–29.

46. Parks EL, Geha PY, Baliki MN, Katz J, Schnitzer TJ, Apkarian AV. Brain activity for chronic knee osteoarthritis: dissociating evoked pain from spontaneous pain. Eur J Pain 2011;15:843.
47. Peat G, McCarney R, Croft P. Knee pain and osteoarthritis in older adults: a review of community burden and current use of primary health care. Ann Rheum Dis 2001;60:91–7.
48. Perrot S, Poiraudeau S, Kabir-Ahmadi M, Rannou F. Correlates of pain intensity in men and women with hip and knee osteoarthritis. Results of a national survey: The French ARTHRIX study. Clin J Pain 2009;25:767–72.
49. Randall LO, Selitto JJ. A method for measurement of analgesic activity on inflamed tissue. Arch Int Pharmacodyn Ther 1957;111:409–19.
50. Rodriguez-Raecke R, Niemeier A, Ihle K, Ruether W, May A. Brain gray matter decrease in chronic pain is the consequence and not the cause of pain. J Neurosci 2009;29:13746–50.
51. Roubille C, Raynauld JP, Abram F, Paiement P, Dorais M, Delorme P, Bessette L, Beaulieu AD, Martel-Pelletier J, Pelletier JP. The presence of meniscal lesions is a strong predictor of neuropathic pain in symptomatic knee osteoarthritis: a cross-sectional pilot study. Arthritis Res Ther 2014;16:507.
52. Ruscheweyh R, Deppe M, Lohmann H, Stehling C, Flöel A, Ringelstein EB, Knecht S. Pain is associated with regional grey matter reduction in the general population. Pain 2011;152:904–11.
53. Stein C, Comisel K, Haimerl E, Yassouridis A, Lehrberger K, Herz A, Peter K. Analgesic effect of intraarticular morphine after arthroscopic knee surgery. N Engl J Med 1991;325:1123–6.
54. Suokas AK, Walsh DA, McWilliams DF, Condon L, Moreton B, Wylde V, Arendt-Nielsen L, Zhang W. QST in painful osteoarthritis: a systematic review and meta-analysis. Osteoarthritis Cartilage 2012;20:1075–85.
55. Taljanovic MS, Graham AR, Benjamin JB, Gmitro AF, Krupinski EA, Schwartz SA, Hunter TB, Resnick DL. Bone marrow edema pattern in advanced hip osteoarthritis: quantitative assessment with magnetic resonance imaging and correlation with clinical examination, radiographic findings, and histopathology. Skeletal Radiol. 2008;37:423–31.
56. Thakur M, Dawes JM, McMahon SB. Genomics of pain in osteoarthritis. Osteoarthritis Cartilage. 2013;21:1374–82.
57. Thompson SWN, Dray A, McCarson KE, Krause JE, Urban L. Nerve growth factor induces mechanical allodynia associated with novel A fibre-evoked spinal reflex activity and enhanced neurokinin-1 receptor activation in the rat. Pain 1995;62:219–32.
58. Timmermans EJ, van der Pas S, Schaap LA, Sánchez-Martínez M, Zambon S, Peter R, Pedersen NL, Dennison EM, Denkinger M, Castell MV, et al. Self-perceived weather sensitivity and joint pain in older people with osteoarthritis in six European countries: results from the European Project on OSteoArthritis (EPOSA). BMC Musculoskelet Disord 2014;15:66.
59. Torres L, Dunlop DD, Peterfy C, Guermazi A, Prasad P, Hayes KW, Song J, Cahue S, Chang A, Marshall M, Sharma L. The relationship between specific

tissue lesions and pain severity in persons with knee osteoarthritis. Osteoarthritis Cartilage 2006;14:1033–40.

60. Woolhead G, Gooberman-Hill R, Dieppe P, Hawker G. Night pain in hip and knee osteoarthritis: a focus group study. Arthritis Care Res (Hoboken) 2010;62:944–9.
61. Wylde V, Palmer S, Learmonth I, Dieppe P. Test–retest reliability of quantitative sensory testing in knee osteoarthritis and healthy participants. Osteoarthritis Cartilage 2011;19:655–8.
62. Zhang RX, Ren K, Dubner R. Osteoarthritis pain mechanisms: basic studies in animal models. Osteoarthritis Cartilage 2013;21:1308–15.

CHAPTER 10

# Exercise Therapy: An Important Pain Reliever in Knee Osteoarthritis

*Søren T. Skou, Lars Arendt-Nielsen, and Ewa M. Roos*

Osteoarthritis (OA), a common cause of knee joint pain, is a worldwide significant contributor to functional disability. The prevalence of painful knee OA has doubled in women and tripled in men during the last 20 years [9] and is expected to increase substantially in the future. Since no cure exists for knee OA, the focus of current treatments is to improve symptoms and prevent further progression of the disease.

On the basis of the research results from the past 25 years, the management of the disease is undergoing a paradigm shift toward early treatment and prevention, reflected in the recommendations from international organizations such as the Osteoarthritis Research Society International (OARSI) [7]. OARSI recommends that first-line treatment, consisting of education, exercise therapy, and weight loss (if needed), is offered to all patients with knee OA, while other nonsurgical treatments (second-line treatment), such as knee brace and pain killers, can be added if first-line treatment does not result in adequate pain relief [7]. Surgical treatment should be considered only after a comprehensive nonsurgical treatment of sufficient dose and length (third-line treatment; Fig. 10-1) [10].

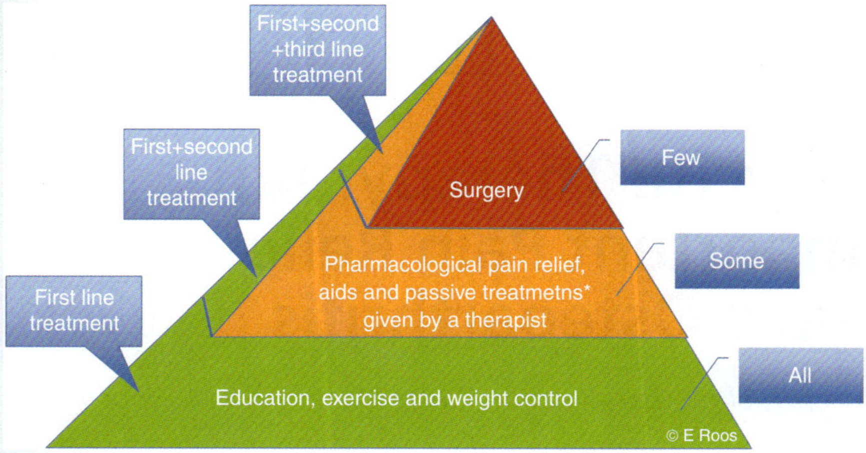


**FIGURE 10-1** Osteoarthritis treatment pyramid. All patients should be offered first-line treatment, while only some need second-line treatment and a still smaller percentage will need third-line treatment. *Passive treatment represents manual therapy, acupuncture, and other treatments given by a therapist that do not require an active effort by the patient. Only if first-line treatment is not sufficient in controlling/reducing the symptoms, second-line treatment, and after that third-line treatment, should be considered. (From Roos and Juhl [10].)

This chapter is about exercise therapy as treatment of pain and disability in knee OA, focusing on the potency of exercise therapy to reduce pain and improve function at all stages of knee OA severity. Furthermore, it will cover issues important for successful pain relief and improvement in function from exercise therapy and the underlying mechanisms causing reduction of pain in patients with knee OA. Lastly, the chapter will address the effects of combining exercise therapy with other nonsurgical treatments and the challenges and possible solutions when implementing treatment recommendations in clinical practice.

## THE EFFECTS OF EXERCISE THERAPY ON PAIN AND FUNCTION

As with several other chronic diseases, the evidence for the benefits of exercise therapy on patient symptoms is substantial. Based on findings from accumulated evidence from the approximately 50 randomized controlled trials (RCTs) conducted in the last 25 years, it is unlikely that future trials will change the conclusion that exercise therapy is effective in reducing pain and improving function in patients with knee OA [6]. Fig. 10-2 presents the effect sizes from meta-analyses of RCTs [6, 7] for improvement in pain and function for some of the most frequently applied first- and second-line treatments. Even though different control treatments have been applied, exercise therapy seems to be the most potent of all nonsurgical treatments in reducing pain and improving function [6, 7]. Compared with the most common pain killers, acetaminophen (paracetamol) and nonsteroidal anti-inflammatory drugs (NSAIDs), exercise therapy is two to three times more effective in reducing pain [6, 7]. At the same time, both paracetamol and NSAIDs are associated with an increased risk of serious adverse events [7], while adverse events, such as delayed onset muscle soreness, pain, and swelling, related to exercise therapy are uncommon, mild, and temporary, even in patients with severe knee OA [1, 20]. This highlights the feasibility and importance of exercise therapy in the treatment of knee OA.

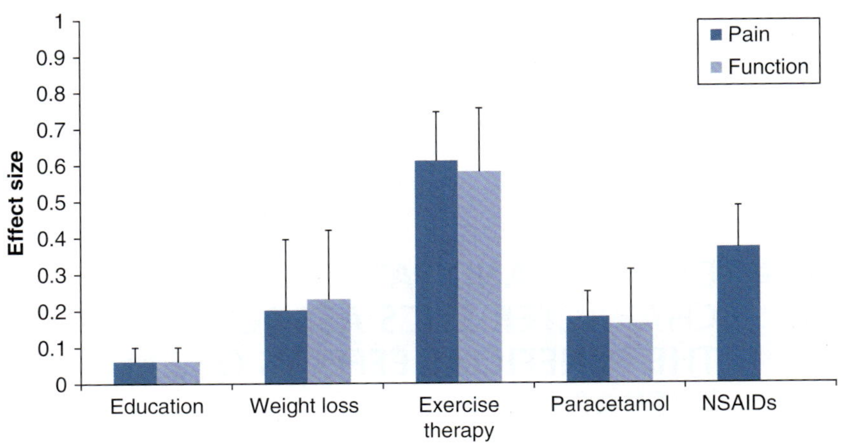


**FIGURE 10-2** Effect sizes for the treatment of knee osteoarthritis (based on meta-analyses of randomized controlled trials [RCTs] [6, 7]). A larger effect size (standardized mean difference [SMD]) indicates a larger effect. SMDs can be clinically interpreted as ≥0.2, small; ≥0.5, moderate; and ≥0.8, large. Error bars indicate upper limit of the 95% CI.

## DISEASE SEVERITY AND EXERCISE THERAPY

The discrepancy between symptomatic (pain) and radiographic OA severity is well proven and largest in population-based samples. Previous studies have demonstrated that the pain-relieving effect of both exercise therapy [6] and other nonsurgical treatments [12] is similar regardless of OA severity as evaluated by radiography. Similarly, exercise therapy is also feasible and effective for pain relief in those with moderate and severe symptomatic knee OA eligible for total knee replacement (TKR) [16, 19], and baseline knee pain is not associated with the size of pain relief from exercise therapy [6]. A recent high-quality RCT in patients with knee OA eligible for TKR demonstrated that TKR in combination with nonsurgical treatment (neuromuscular exercise, education, diet, insoles, and pain medication) was more efficacious in improving pain and function but was associated with more serious adverse events than the nonsurgical treatment alone [16]. However, the patients randomized to nonsurgical treatment alone had clinically relevant pain relief, and 74% did not undergo TKR within 1 year [16]. These findings highlight the potency of nonsurgical treatment, including exercise, in the treatment of patients with knee OA at all stages of disease severity. Since knee OA can be diagnosed from clinical criteria, and since only 0.5% of knee radiographs reveal treatment-changing pathologies [17], clinicians can confidently refer the patient to exercise therapy regardless of radiographic and symptomatic OA severity.

## EXERCISE AND PATIENT CHARACTERISTICS ASSOCIATED WITH THE BENEFICIAL EFFECTS OF EXERCISE THERAPY

A wide range of exercise therapy programs has been applied in the approximately 50 RCTs published on exercise therapy in knee OA [6]. In general, these exercise therapy programs can be grouped into three overarching types: aerobic exercise (focusing on improving cardiorespiratory fitness), resistance exercise (focusing on improving muscle strength), and performance exercise (focusing on improving the performance of a specific activity). These overarching types of exercise therapy reveal similar efficacy with effect sizes (standardized mean difference [SMD]) of 0.67 and 0.56 for aerobic exercise, 0.62 and 0.60 for resistance exercise, and 0.48 and 0.56 for performance exercise for improvements of pain and function, respectively. It is important to recognize that this does not mean that the choice of exercise type is less significant when treating the individual patient, as several studies have identified subgroups of patients with knee OA benefitting more from one type of exercise therapy than the other. One example is from a recent exploratory analysis from an RCT showing that patients with a visually observable varus thrust (dynamic worsening or abrupt onset of varus malalignment of the knee during the stance phase of gait) and nonobese patients improved more in pain from neuromuscular exercise aiming at improving functional stability of the joint than from quadriceps strengthening. Obese patients, on the other hand, benefitted more from quadriceps training [3]. Identifying subgroups of patients more likely to benefit from specific treatments is a major focus in the current OA research aiming at developing individualized treatment of the patients based on specific characteristics and thereby further boosting individual treatment effects.

While three or more exercise therapy sessions per week are more efficacious in improving pain (but not function) than less than two sessions per week, intensity and duration of the exercise therapy sessions seem less important for the treatment efficacy in patients with knee OA [6]. However, it seems reasonable that a sufficient exercise dosage (defined by frequency, intensity, and duration) and increased levels of progression over time are important for optimal effects from exercise therapy.

The number of supervised exercise therapy sessions is of importance for the outcome. Results from a meta-analysis showed that 12 or more supervised sessions were nearly twice as effective as less than 12 sessions in improving both pain (SMD: 0.46 vs. 0.28) and function (SMD: 0.45 vs. 0.23) [4]. This has recently been confirmed by another meta-analysis demonstrating improved efficacy in reducing pain with more supervised exercise therapy sessions [6]. Ongoing supervision and feedback are important, not only because of the larger improvements from more supervised sessions, but also because of the educational elements embedded in the interaction with the physical therapist supervising the patient.

## EXERCISE THERAPY ADHERENCE: A KEY COMPONENT FOR LONG-TERM IMPROVEMENTS IN PAIN AND FUNCTION

Adherence has been highlighted as one of the most important components of a successful outcome of treatment with exercise therapy because of the dose–response relationship seen in patients with knee OA pain [20]. At the same time, the beneficial effects from exercise therapy are short lived and only last as long as the patient continues to exercise. Therefore, it is important that the patients undergo proper patient education. Despite a small effect size (Fig. 10-2) [7], potentially explained by how the effect was measured (pain and function were measured rather than the efficacy of education on adherence to treatment, anxiety, self-efficacy, etc.), education is an important aspect of the treatment because of the pivotal role of the patient in the treatment of knee OA pain and disability. Exercise therapy (and other treatments requiring the patient to be active) will only be beneficial if the patient is committed to actively engage in the treatment. Therefore, a concurrent educational aspect teaching the patient about knee OA symptoms and risk factors, pain mechanisms and etiology, self-help tools, and the importance of the lifelong continuation of treatment for a chronic disease such as OA is essential for adherence and long-term pain relief and functional improvement.

Involving the patient in a shared decision-making process is crucial. To ensure high adherence, potential barriers and facilitators to exercise should be identified and addressed at the initiation of the exercise therapy program. Furthermore, to improve long-term adherence, exercise should be integrated into daily life of the individual patient in parallel with a period of supervised exercise therapy allowing for monitoring, progression of exercises, and managing any fears related to exercising and being physically active.

Recently, web-based applications have been developed to enable exercise therapy to be self-supervised or even prescribed, supervised, and adjusted by an intelligent computer system or a physical therapist based on specific characteristics entered by or transferred from the patient or using videoconferencing. It is likely that web-based applications will be increasingly popular in the future, and they hold promising perspectives as a supplement to regular face-to-face supervision of exercise therapy to improve adherence to exercise. However, studies investigating web-based exercise therapy in addition to and/or in direct comparison with face-to-face supervision are required to elucidate the role of web-based exercise therapy in the treatment of knee OA.

## WHY DOES EXERCISE THERAPY REDUCE PAIN IN KNEE OSTEOARTHRITIS?

While the evidence for the efficacy of the exercise therapy to reduce pain and improve function in patients with knee OA is strong [18], surprisingly little is known about why exercise therapy reduces pain [11]. Potential explanations are often given in the introduction or discussion sections of papers in the field, but few of them have actual evidence to support these explanations. Fig. 10-3 depicts some of the mechanisms previously proposed to influence the pain reduction from exercise therapy in patients with knee OA. A recent systematic review tried to identify possible mediators of the improvement in pain and function from exercise therapy based on physiological mechanisms measured alongside pain and function in the individual studies [11]. The systematic review identified increased upper leg muscle strength, decreased extension impairments, and improvements in proprioception as possible mediators of improvements in pain and function based on a large percentage of studies showing a significant improvement in these physiological mechanisms compared to no change or inconclusive change [11].

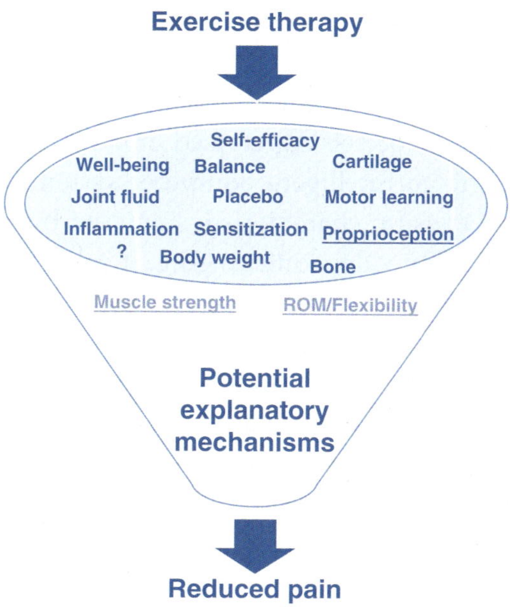


**FIGURE 10-3** Mechanisms that could explain the pain reduction from exercise therapy in patients with knee osteoarthritis. The mechanisms described are not exhaustive, but can be regarded as potential mechanisms explaining the pain reduction from exercise therapy either alone or in combination with other mechanisms. Mechanisms underlined have been identified as possible mediators of improvements in pain from exercise therapy [11]. ROM, range of motion.

Exercise therapy in combination with other nonsurgical treatments reduces pain not only in the OA knee, but also in other body parts. A predefined ancillary analysis from an RCT demonstrated that a group of patients with knee OA not eligible for TKR had a larger reduction in the number of body sites, with pain following the nonsurgical treatment compared with a group of patients receiving information alone [13]. This could be related to systemic anti-inflammatory effects from exercise therapy and/or improvements in well-being and other psychosocial mechanisms. In the same study, the authors investigated the effects of the nonsurgical treatment on sensitization, which is known to be an important pain mechanism in knee OA. In the group receiving nonsurgical treatment, the proportion with diffuse knee pain was reduced, and at the same time, the knee pain intensity was reduced more than in the group receiving information alone. This concurrent improvement in pain and sensitization indicates that sensitization could be another explanatory mechanism for the improvement in pain from exercise therapy. However, both groups of the study improved in other measures, reflecting localized sensitization (peripheral sensitization: pressure pain thresholds [PPTs] from the knee) and spreading sensitization (central sensitization: PPTs from the lower leg and forearm), with no between group differences [13]. This leaves sensitization as a potential explanatory mechanism for the effects of exercise therapy on pain, which requires further investigation. Importantly, since the nonsurgical treatment also included other treatments, such as patient education, teaching the patient about pain mechanisms and how to deal with the pain, it cannot be concluded that the effects of the study were based on exercise therapy alone [13].

Finally, it is important to recognize that the improvement in pain from exercise therapy is probably not caused by a single mechanism, but should instead be regarded as a complex interaction between both physiological and psychosocial mechanisms. At the same time, it is likely that these mechanisms differ between individual patients, yet again highlighting that exercise therapy should be individualized (e.g., exercise type, intensity, and level of difficulty) based on patient characteristics such as those described in the section on exercise and patient characteristics associated with the beneficial effects from the exercise therapy above.

## COMBINED EFFECT OF EXERCISE THERAPY AND OTHER NONSURGICAL TREATMENTS ON PAIN AND FUNCTION

By combining exercise therapy with other recommended nonsurgical treatments, the effects on pain and function can be improved even further. While two previous RCTs have investigated the long-term efficacy of a combination of two of the recommended treatments as compared with usual care in patients with knee OA [5, 8], a recent RCT combined neuromuscular exercise, education, diet, insoles, and pain medication (recommended first- and second-line treatments from Fig. 10-1), individualized to the needs and characteristics (such as mediolateral knee motion, weight, and pain intensity) of patients with knee OA pain [14]. The Arthritis, Diet, and Activity Promotion Trial combined exercise therapy and weight loss and demonstrated improvements in the treatment group in pain and function of 30% and 24%, respectively [8], while the study combining first- and second-line treatments found larger improvements in pain (36%) and function (37%) in the treatment group at the long-term follow-up (12 months)[14]. The Enabling Self-Management and Coping of Arthritic Knee Pain through Exercise Trial combining exercise therapy and education found that even though pain and function improved more in the treatment group immediately after the intervention, these improvements were not sustained at long-term follow-up [5]. After adjustment, the mean difference between groups in function was approximately 5 on a 0–100 scale at the long-term follow-up [5]. The study combining first- and second-line treatments demonstrated that the effects on pain and function were sustained at the long-term follow-up, with difference in function between treatment groups being twice as large (adjusted difference of 11.2 on a 0–100 scale) [14]. The authors suggest that the larger improvements in the study combining first- and second-line treatments could be attributed to differences in the interventions given in the studies, in particular a more focused neuromuscular exercise program of sufficient dose and length and the combination of exercise therapy, education, and, if required, diet, insoles, and pain medication delivered in an individualized fashion.

## IMPLEMENTATION OF EXERCISE THERAPY IN CLINICAL PRACTICE TO IMPROVE PAIN AND FUNCTION IN THE POPULATION

Despite the strong evidence supporting the efficacy of exercise therapy and the international recommendations highlighting exercise therapy as first-line treatment in patients with painful knee OA, the uptake in clinical practice is suboptimal. A systematic review and meta-analysis summarizing studies assessing the quality of care in OA using quality indicators found pass rates, defined as the percentage of patients receiving appropriate care according to guidelines, of only 36.1% (95% CI, 27.8–44.7%) for nonpharmacological treatment of OA [2]. This low level of patients receiving appropriate care underlines that initiatives aimed at implementing evidence-based guidelines for the treatment of knee OA in clinical practice are important to facilitate high quality care of patients with knee OA in the population. However, implementing clinical guidelines in clinical practice represents a major problem of modern health care, and a range of barriers needs to be addressed to ensure successful implementation. The literature stresses that to be successful in putting research into action in clinical practice, a comprehensive approach fit to the specific target groups and settings is needed.

In Denmark, such an initiative was developed in 2013, aimed at implementing clinical guidelines for the treatment of knee and hip OA into clinical care [15]. The initiative is called Good Life with Osteoarthritis in Denmark (GLA:D) and consists of three parts:

1. A 2-day course for physical therapists teaching them to deliver OA care in accordance with clinical guidelines.
2. Eight weeks of patient education (three 90-min sessions) and neuromuscular exercise (12 supervised exercise therapy sessions) for patients with OA symptoms from the knee and/or hip.
3. The national GLA:D registry for data collection and evaluation of results (both objectively measured, therapist-reported and patient-reported outcomes) at baseline, 3 and 12 months.

So far more than 12000 patients with knee and/or hip OA have received education and exercise therapy through GLA:D. The annual report of 2015 presents results from the 9827 patients who had been enrolled until 31 December 2015, of which 5846 patients had undergone the 3-month follow-up and 2149 the 12-month follow-up [14]. After 3 months, the pain was reduced by 28% and after 12 months by 28% compared with before GLA:D in patients with knee OA. Before GLA:D, 56% were using pain medication (paracetamol, NSAIDs, or opioids) because of their painful knee, while only 37% were using it after 3 months. Furthermore, sick leave was reduced from 30% of the patients related to the labor market being on sick leave before GLA:D because of their knee or hip to 20% being on sick leave after 12 months [15]. While it is important to recognize that data are coming from a registry, without the control group and rigorous research setting of an RCT, the results from clinical practice are encouraging and hold promising perspectives easily transferable to other countries to improve the quality of care in patients with painful knee OA.

## CONCLUSIONS

Exercise therapy is the most efficacious of all nonsurgical treatments of painful knee OA, no matter the severity of the disease as evaluated by joint degeneration and pain. Together with education, exercise therapy should be offered to all patients with painful knee OA as early as possible to prevent progression of the symptoms. The exercise therapy should be tailored to the individual based on patient characteristics (such as weight, pain intensity, and mediolateral knee motion), and strategies to improve long-term adherence should be implemented to ensure continuation of lifelong exercise. Implementation of evidence-based exercise therapy in clinical practice represents a key challenge in future health care to improve the quality of care on a population level. Using a comprehensive approach fitted to the specific target groups and settings, initiatives delivering education and exercise on a nationwide level can overcome barriers and successfully implement clinical guidelines for the treatment of knee OA.

## REFERENCES

1. Ageberg E, Link A, Roos EM. Feasibility of neuromuscular training in patients with severe hip or knee OA: the individualized goal-based NEMEX-TJR training program. BMC Musculoskelet Disord 2010;11:126.
2. Basedow M, Esterman A. Assessing appropriateness of osteoarthritis care using quality indicators: a systematic review. J Eval Clin Pract 2015;21:782–9.

3. Bennell KL, Dobson F, Roos EM, Skou ST, Hodges P, Wrigley TV, Kyriakides M, Metcalf B, Hunt MA, Hinman RS. The influence of biomechanical characteristics on pain and function outcomes from exercise in medial knee osteoarthritis and varus malalignment: exploratory analyses from a randomised controlled trial. Arthritis Care Res (Hoboken) 2015;67:1281–8.
4. Fransen M, McConnell S. Exercise for osteoarthritis of the knee. Cochrane Database Syst Rev 2008;CD004376.
5. Hurley MV, Walsh NE, Mitchell H, Nicholas J, Patel A. Long-term outcomes and costs of an integrated rehabilitation program for chronic knee pain: a pragmatic, cluster randomized, controlled trial. Arthritis Care Res (Hoboken) 2012;64:238–47.
6. Juhl C, Christensen R, Roos EM, Zhang W, Lund H. Impact of exercise type and dose on pain and disability in knee osteoarthritis: a systematic review and meta-regression analysis of randomized controlled trials. Arthritis Rheumatol 2014;66:622–36. doi:10 1002/art 38290.
7. McAlindon TE, Bannuru RR, Sullivan MC, Arden NK, Berenbaum F, Bierma-Zeinstra SM, Hawker GA, Henrotin Y, Hunter DJ, Kawaguchi H, et al. OARSI guidelines for the non-surgical management of knee osteoarthritis. Osteoarthritis Cartilage 2014;22:363–88.
8. Messier SP, Loeser RF, Miller GD, Morgan TM, Rejeski WJ, Sevick MA, Ettinger WH Jr, Pahor M, Williamson JD. Exercise and dietary weight loss in overweight and obese older adults with knee osteoarthritis: the Arthritis, Diet, and Activity Promotion Trial. Arthritis Rheum 2004;50:1501–10.
9. Nguyen US, Zhang Y, Zhu Y, Niu J, Zhang B, Felson DT. Increasing prevalence of knee pain and symptomatic knee osteoarthritis: survey and cohort data. Ann Intern Med 2011;155:725–32.
10. Roos EM, Juhl CB. Osteoarthritis 2012 year in review: rehabilitation and outcomes. Osteoarthritis Cartilage 2012;20:1477–83.
11. Runhaar J, Luijsterburg P, Dekker J, Bierma-Zeinstra SM. Identifying potential working mechanisms behind the positive effects of exercise therapy on pain and function in osteoarthritis; a systematic review. Osteoarthritis Cartilage 2015;23:1071–82.
12. Skou ST, Derosche CA, Andersen MM, Rathleff MS, Simonsen O. Nonoperative treatment improves pain irrespective of radiographic severity—a cohort study of 1,414 patients with knee osteoarthritis. Acta Orthop 2015;86:1–6.
13. Skou ST, Rasmussen S, Laursen MB, Rathleff MS, Arendt-Nielsen L, Simonsen O, Roos EM. The efficacy of non-surgical treatment on pain and sensitization in patients with knee osteoarthritis: a pre-defined ancillary analysis from a randomized controlled trial. Osteoarthritis Cartilage 2016;24:108–16.
14. Skou ST, Rasmussen S, Laursen MB, Rathleff MS, Arendt-Nielsen L, Simonsen O, Roos EM. The efficacy of 12 weeks non-surgical treatment for patients not eligible for total knee replacement: a randomized controlled trial with 1-year follow-up. Osteoarthritis Cartilage 2015;23:1465–75.
15. Skou ST, Roos EM. GLA:D Annual Report 2015. 2016;3.

16. Skou ST, Roos EM, Laursen MB, Rathleff MS, Arendt-Nielsen L, Simonsen O, Rasmussen S. A randomized controlled trial of total knee replacement. N Engl J Med 2015;373:1597–1606.
17. Skou ST, Thomsen H, Simonsen OH. The value of routine radiography in patients with knee osteoarthritis consulting primary health care: a study of agreement. Eur J Gen Pract 2014;20:10–16.
18. Uthman OA, van der Windt DA, Jordan JL, Dziedzic KS, Healey EL, Peat GM, Foster NE. Exercise for lower limb osteoarthritis: systematic review incorporating trial sequential analysis and network meta-analysis. BMJ 2013;347:f5555.
19. Villadsen A, Overgaard S, Holsgaard-Larsen A, Christensen R, Roos EM. Immediate efficacy of neuromuscular exercise in patients with severe osteoarthritis of the hip or knee: a secondary analysis from a randomized controlled trial. J Rheumatol 2014;41:1385–94.
20. Wang SY, Olson-Kellogg B, Shamliyan TA, Choi JY, Ramakrishnan R, Kane RL. Physical therapy interventions for knee pain secondary to osteoarthritis: a systematic review. Ann Intern Med 2012;157:632–44.

CHAPTER 11

# Chronic Pain after Joint Surgery

*Kristian Kjær Petersen and Lars Arendt-Nielsen*

In the United States, the economic consequence of lost working days due to chronic pain is estimated to be between $560 and $635 billion per year, in which a proportion is due to chronic postoperative pain following joint replacement surgery. Many patients end up on social security as a consequence of lost or reduced ability to work. A large demand for more efficient and safe drugs and applicable medical devices for pain prevention and treatment thus continues to drive the pain management market.

Chronic postoperative pain is defined by the International Association for the Study of Pain (IASP) as persistent pain 6 months after surgery. Two major joint replacements are total knee replacement (TKR) and total hip replacement (THR) surgeries, and this chapter focuses on the prevalence of chronic postoperative pain after TKR and THR surgery in knee osteoarthritis (KOA) and hip osteoarthritis (HOA) and covers the potential preoperative risk factors for the development of chronic postoperative pain (Fig. 11-1).

## CHRONIC POSTOPERATIVE PAIN

A debate regarding the prevalence of chronic postoperative pain after TKR and THR surgery is ongoing. Beswick et al. [5] concluded based

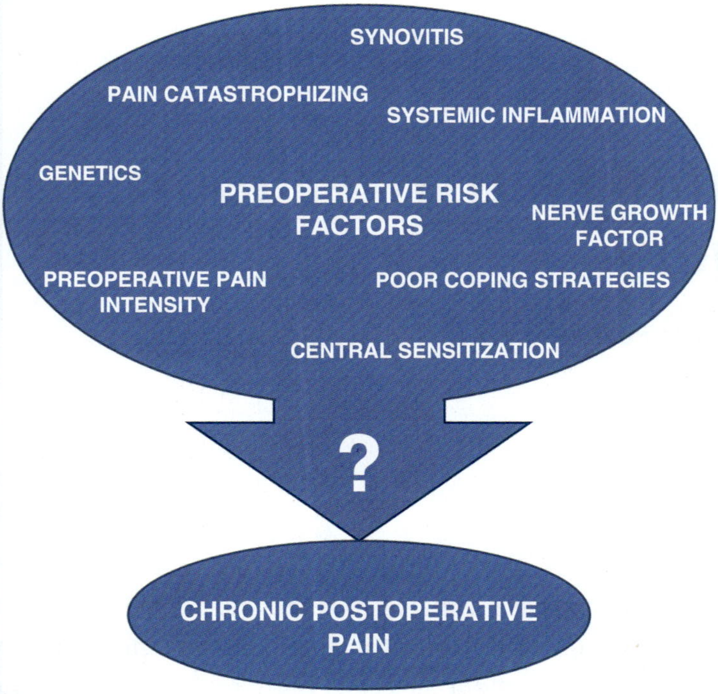


**FIGURE 11-1** Potential preoperative risk factors for the development of chronic postoperative pain.

on a meta-analysis that the overall proportion of chronic postoperative pain after TKR and THR surgery was ~20% and 10%, respectively. Currently, there is no definitive explanation as to why some patients develop chronic postoperative pain while others have a pain-free recovery.

## Pain after Revision Surgery

Eighty percent to 90% of total knee arthroplasty (TKA)/total hip arthroplasty (THA) revision surgeries are performed because of pain, aseptic loosing, infection, instability, and stiffness. Up to 50% of the patients following re-TKR surgery will continue to have chronic postoperative pain [22], and re-TKR surgery is associated with a high risk of multiple re-TKR surgeries [7].

### Treatment of Osteoarthritis

Several pharmacological and nonpharmacological treatment guidelines are available for OA. Increasing evidence suggests that exercise and body mass index reduction will decrease pain in patients with joint pain. However, a recent study showed that joint replacement surgery is still superior compared with exercise in patients with severe KOA, although the exercise may postpone surgery [29]. The current end-stage treatment for severe KOA or HOA is TKR or THR surgery, respectively. The amount of THR is predicted to increase by almost 200% and TKR by almost 700% by 2030 in the United States [17].

TKR and THR have a low rate of technical errors, but still 20% of TKR patients and 10% of THR patients are rendered into chronic postoperative pain [5]. Few attempts have been made to subgroup OA patients; however, these subgroups have shown different degeneration of the joint, different sensory pain profiles [8], and different outcomes after total joint replacement surgery [21, 33]. With the rising number of treatable patients and the risk of developing chronic postoperative pain, the industry, the researchers, and the health care sector have to develop new preoperative prediction methods for personalized treatment to comply with this growing problem.

## OSTEOARTHRITIS AS A MODEL FOR THE DEVELOPMENT OF CHRONIC POSTOPERATIVE PAIN

Preoperative pain intensity [15, 21], comorbidities [15], sensitization [2, 21, 33], genetic factors [10], inflammation [9], and psychological profiles [3] are factors that have been linked to the outcomes after surgery.

OA is recognized as a disease involving all joint tissues, but the specific pain mechanisms in OA are largely unknown. The diagnosis of KOA is based on a combination of symptomatic pain and stiffness and radiographic assessments such as the Kellgren and Lawrence (KL) score, which is a measure for the loss of cartilage. Interestingly, in the individual patient, there is little correlation between the pain intensity in KOA and the KL score, suggesting that other factors than cartilage damage are involved. Studies have shown that specific groups of patients with OA characterized by high pain but low radiological severity seem to be highly pain sensitive [1, 8], and low radiological severity before TKR has been linked to low functional level after surgery [25].

Preoperative pain intensity has been shown to be a clinical predictor for the development of chronic pain, and the acute postoperative pain is correlated with the development of chronic postoperative pain [15]. In addition, higher analgesia consumption in the acute operative phase has been shown to be risk factors [15].

In recent years, the role of the synovium and synovitis in OA has attracted increased attention. A systematic review from 2011 [35] concluded that synovitis is associated with knee OA pain. Interestingly, the synovial membrane is not completely removed during, for example, TKR, despite ongoing synovitis, which could be a reason for ongoing pain after joint replacement. However, further research is needed to evaluate this.

## Nerve Growth Factor

When a nerve is cut, the Schwann cells, and other cells in the area of injury, produce the nerve growth factor (NGF) [31]. NGF is critical for normal neuronal development, and withdrawal of NGF or blocking its receptor results in decreased pain sensitivity, and experimental injection of NGF leads to increased pain sensitivity. The concept nerve sprouting, which is a result of increased NGF release, has been observed in cancer-induced animal bone pain models, which increased generation of nociceptive fibers [13]. It is hypothesized that increased NGF release due to surgical trauma could lead to nerve sprouting, which in turn could lead to chronic postoperative pain.

Inhibition of NGF by monoclonal antibodies has been demonstrated to reduce the pain and increase the function and well-being of individuals with symptomatic OA. The magnitude of this response provides evidence that inhibition of NGF-mediated processes is potent means of suppressing pain. However, side effects, including the high incidence of reversible abnormalities of peripheral sensation, have hampered the development of anti-NGF drugs [26].

Sensitization of nociceptive fibers has been widely studied in the last decade with the focus on comparison between the healthy and OA-affected tissue, and, recently, also on the prognostic information in preoperative screening using quantitative sensory testing (QST).

## Sensitization of the Nervous System

QST is a tool for monitoring and diagnosing pain processing and its alterations in patients. It has been widely used to study peripheral and central sensitization in patients with musculoskeletal pain [2]. The concept of QST is to use standardized, defined stimuli under standardized conditions, while the subject rates the stimulus on the basis of the experienced pain. The use of multiple stimulus modalities with different intensities or one prolonged stimuli with increasing intensity makes it possible to construct stimulus–response relationships, which characterize the subject's pain sensitivity. Hyperalgesia can objectively be quantified by a leftward shift in the stimulus–response curve compared with a healthy control subject.

QST aims to give an insight into the pain mechanisms compared, for example, with the simple visual analog scale (VAS). However, QST is time-consuming and requires a training of the subject in a reliable and accurate rating of the pain stimuli. Combining different stimulation techniques allows for a more complete quantification of the state of the nervous system [2].

Pain intensity and duration of OA have been found to be associated with the degree of sensitization [2]. Pre- and acute postoperative treatment with pregabalin seems to inhibit the development of chronic postoperative neuropathic pain after joint replacement [6], which may indicate that the sensitization plays a key role in determining the outcome of joint replacement surgery. A recent review concludes that increased pain duration is associated with a higher degree of central sensitization and that central sensitization is highly involved in the pain of OA [2].

OA is associated with local and widespread hyperalgesia compared with controls, which is improved after pain-free joint replacement surgery [2]. A higher degree of general sensitization (i.e., around the knee) has been shown to be related to higher levels of pain [2], disability and poorer quality of life [12], and poorer outcome after joint replacement surgery [20]. Preoperative widespread hyperalgesia has been linked to the development of chronic postoperative pain following THR [33].

Increased facilitated temporal summation, as a measure of central integrative mechanisms induced by a sequence of stimuli with the same intensity where a progressive increase in pain occurs, has been documented in OA patients compared with controls [2]. Recently, preoperative temporal summation has been shown to predict the development of chronic postoperative pain following TKR surgery [21].

Dysfunctional endogenous nociceptive inhibition, measured as impaired conditioning pain modulation (CPM), has been documented in patients with OA, which is restored after pain-free joint replacement [2]. Preoperative impaired CPM has been associated with development of chronic postoperative pain after thoracotomy [34] and abdominal surgery [32], but no association has been documented in patients undergoing total joint replacement.

Sensitization seems to be normalized in patients with a pain-free recovery when comparing pre- and postoperative QST measurements [2]. However, patients with ongoing pain after, for example, primary TKR surgery can be offered revision TKA surgery (re-TKA), but re-TKR is involved with high risk of a poor outcome. Patients with pain after re-TKR surgery show widespread hyperalgesia, facilitated temporal summation, and lower CPM compared with patients with no pain after re-TKR surgery [27]. Facilitated temporal summation is more predominant in patients with widespread hyperalgesia after re-TKR surgery compared with KOA patients before primary TKR surgery [28]. This could indicate a continued nociceptive drive, despite the removal of the OA-affected joint, further indicating that sensitization could play a key role in the chronification of postoperative pain. This suggests that sensitization should be considered before re-TKR surgery.

Limited evidence indicates that the thermal sensitivity is changed in patients with OA compared with healthy controls [16].

The current working hypothesis of different sensory profiles is illustrated in Fig. 11-2, in which a patient with lower preoperative sensitization will undergo an increase in sensitization in the acute postoperative phase but return to a low sensitization state after pain-free recovery in the postoperative phase. Also, illustrated in Fig. 11-2 is the patient with higher preoperative sensitization, who will also have an increase in acute postoperative sensitization and an increased postoperative sensitization, which is linked with chronic postoperative pain [2, 21, 33].

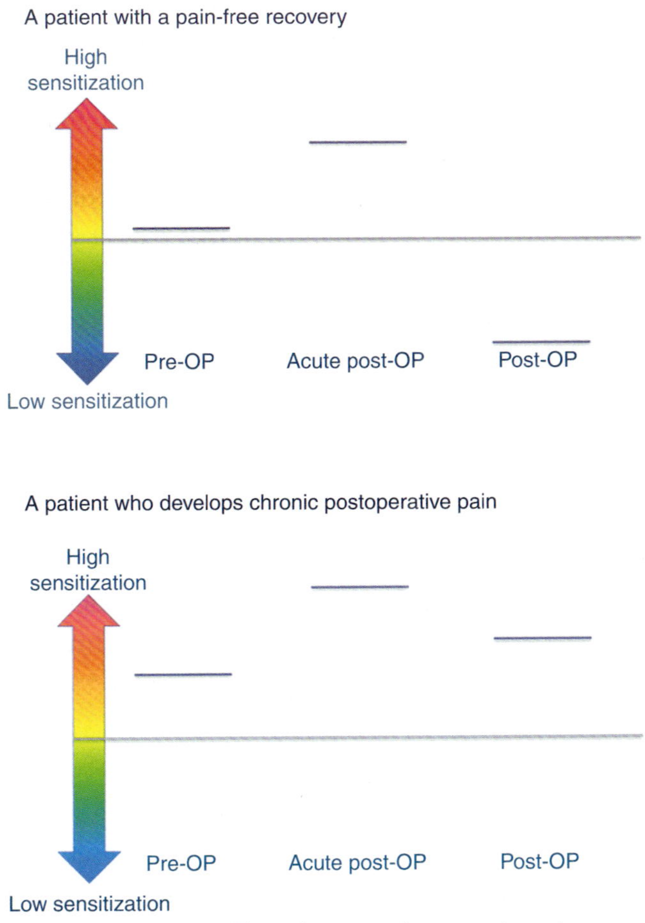


**FIGURE 11-2** Sensitization profiles of two patients undergoing total joint replacement in the preoperative (pre-OP) acute postoperative (acute post-OP) and chronic postoperative (post-OP) phases.

The transition between the acute postoperative phase and the chronic postoperative phase is not completely understood.

## Genetics and Joint Pain

Genetic epidemiology is the study of genetic factors that influence the dynamics of disease in populations. Studies have shown that genetics can influence the risk of developing OA and the progression in the different stages of OA. Obesity, gender, age, skeletal shape, and bone mass are examples of genetic factors, which can influence the progression of OA. Low age is linked with a more vigorous neoplastic response, and gender differences have been shown in regards to pain modulation, and therefore, they are classified as risk factors for postoperative pain after joint replacement. More women than men are diagnosed with OA [30], and women in general report higher postoperative pain than men [15].

Untreated comorbidities and additional pain problems to the primary reason for surgery should be identified and treated, if possible, to minimize the risk of postoperative chronic pain [15].

Less known examples of genetic factors are genetically increased pain sensitivity or genes encoding for, for example, interleukins (IL). The catechol-*O*-methyltransferase (*COMT* gene) has been shown to be associated with hip pain in patients with HOA, and the gene coding for IL-6 has been positively correlated with osteolysis in patients after THA [10]. Other genetic factors include, for example, the single nucleotide polymorphism (SNP) in the *SCN9A* gene (encoding for specific sodium channels), which is associated with increased pain levels if present in OA patients, leading to changed pain thresholds [24].

## Inflammation in Joint Pain

Cytokines are known not only to contribute to the degradation of the joint but also to play an important role in pain generation. In disease-free conditions, the balance between pro- and anti-inflammatory cytokines enables, for example, a stable level of cartilage and does not interfere with pain. In OA, there is an imbalance between these cytokines contributing to the pathophysiology, but generally, anti-inflammatory cytokines have been less studied in the search of OA biomarkers. In particular, IL-10 and IL-4 contribute to the suppression of inflammation in the synovial tissue. IL-2 has been found to be higher in knee OA patients compared with healthy subjects after a 10-year follow-up period [18]. Further, serological levels of IL-2, IL-4, and IL-10 have been detected in OA patients in the early and advanced stages [4].

Recently, it was reported that higher preoperative levels of tumor necrosis factor alpha, matrix metalloproteinase-13 (MMP-13), and IL-6 in synovial fluid were associated with a small improvement in pain 2 years after TKR [9].

### Psychological Factors

During the last decade, depression and anxiety have been studied as a potential underlying mechanism for pain in patients with arthritis. For specific courses of pain, self-efficacy (the belief that one has the ability to control pain) [19], pain catastrophizing (the belief that pain will get worse and that one cannot deal with it) [14], and fear of movement (the belief that movement will generate pain and additional injury) [11] have been studied. A recent review concluded that the preoperative presence of catastrophic thinking and poor coping strategies predicted more postoperative pain, that there was no association between preoperative fear of movement and postoperative pain, and that there is conflicting evidence whether preoperative depressive symptoms and anxiety predict postoperative pain after TKR [3].

## FUTURE FOCUS

Several risk factors for chronic postoperative pain have been identified. This section will deal with limitations in the current literature, on which future research could focus to decrease the risk of patients developing chronic postoperative pain following joint replacement surgery.

## Preoperative Sensitization

Several studies suggest that OA patients are sensitized before joint replacement surgery and normalized after surgery [2]. Accumulating evidence suggests that subdividing patients yields subgroups with different sensory profiles, which will have different outcomes after total joint replacement surgery [22, 33].

As described earlier, drugs designed to block the *N*-methyl-D-aspartate receptors have shown decreased facilitated temporal summation, and drugs that promote the reuptake serotonin and norepinephrine have proven to increase descending pain inhibition, reducing knee pain in patients with KOA. Although these drugs are available, the current selection of drugs is limited, which could explain why central sensitized pain syndromes are often difficult to treat. Drug administration could be targeted at different subgroups of patients based on a preoperative QST screening [23].

## Pain Catastrophizing and Coping Strategies

A recent review concluded that the preoperative presence of catastrophic thinking and poor coping strategies predicted more postoperative pain, that there was no association between preoperative fear of movement and postoperative pain, and that there is conflicting evidence whether preoperative depressive symptoms and anxiety predict postoperative pain after TKR [3]. Studies focusing on preoperative treatment of pain catastrophizing and coping strategies are encouraged.

## Synovitis

Yusuf et al. [35] concluded that inflamed synovium generates pain in patients with OA. Today, the synovium is not completely removed during total joint replacement, and therefore, an ongoing inflammation of the synovium could offer an explanation as to why some patients report chronic postoperative pain. Only limited research has been focused on postoperative synovitis; so further investigations should be welcomed.

## CONCLUSION

Preoperative pain intensity has been shown to be a clinical predictor for the development of chronic pain, and the acute postoperative pain is correlated with the development of chronic postoperative pain. In addition, higher analgesia consumption in the acute operative phase has been shown to be risk factors. Women seem to have a higher risk of chronic postoperative pain, and an association between low age and the development of chronic postoperative pain has been shown.

Preoperative central-acting pain mechanisms have been shown to predict the development of chronic postoperative pain in patients undergoing TKR and THR. Further, patients with a low degree of radiological OA by high pain seem to be highly sensitized, and a low degree of radiological OA has been linked to a lower level of function postoperatively.

A single study has shown that preoperative and acute postoperative treatments with pregabalin seem to inhibit the development of chronic postoperative neuropathic pain in patients undergoing TKR. This further indicates that preoperative sensitization of the nervous system might be connected to the development of postoperative chronic pain.

Pain catastrophizing is described as a maladaptive cognitive style employed by anxiety and depression disorders (negative forecast of future events), and preoperative pain catastrophizing has been shown to be a risk factor for chronic postoperative pain following TKR surgery.

Inflammation can lead to sensitization of the nervous fibers, and a preoperative imbalance of specific cytokines has been linked to the development of chronic postoperative pain after joint replacement.

## REFERENCES

1. Arendt-Nielsen L, Eskehave TN, Egsgaard LL, Petersen KK, Graven-Nielsen T, Hoeck HC, Simonsen O, Siebuhr AS, Karsdal M, Bay-Jensen AC. Association between experimental pain biomarkers and serologic markers in patients with different degrees of painful knee osteoarthritis. Arthritis Rheum 2014;66:3317–26.
2. Arendt-Nielsen L, Skou ST, Nielsen TA, Petersen KK. Altered central sensitization and pain modulation in the CNS in chronic joint pain. Curr Osteoporos Rep 2015:1–10.

3. Baert IA, Lluch E, Mulder T, Nijs J, Noten S, Meeus M. Does pre-surgical central modulation of pain influence outcome after total knee replacement? A systematic review. Osteoarthritis Cartilage 2015;24:213–23.
4. Barker T, Rogers VE, Henriksen VT, Aguirre D, Trawick RH, Rasmussen GL, Momberger NG. Serum cytokines are increased and circulating micronutrients are not altered in subjects with early compared to advanced knee osteoarthritis. Cytokine 2014;68:133–36.
5. Beswick AD, Wylde V, Gooberman-Hill R, Blom A, Dieppe P. What proportion of patients report long-term pain after total hip or knee replacement for osteoarthritis? A systematic review of prospective studies in unselected patients. BMJ Open 2012;2:e000435.
6. Buvanendran A, Kroin JS, Della Valle CJ, Kari M, Moric M, Tuman KJ. Perioperative oral pregabalin reduces chronic pain after total knee arthroplasty: a prospective, randomized, controlled trial. Anesth Analg 2010;110:199–207.
7. Davidson D, de Steiger R, Graves S, Tomkins A. Australian orthopaedic association national joint replacement rigister; hip and knee arthroplasty: annual report 2010. Annual report. Adelaide: Australian Orthopaedic Association; 2010.
8. Finan PH, Buenaver LF, Bounds SC, Hussain S, Park RJ, Haque UJ, Campbell CM, Haythornthwaite JA, Edwards RR, Smith MT. Discordance between pain and radiographic severity in knee osteoarthritis: findings from quantitative sensory testing of central sensitization. Arthritis Rheum 2013;65:363–72.
9. Gandhi R, Santone D, Takahashi M, Dessouki O, Mahomed NN. Inflammatory predictors of ongoing pain 2 years following knee replacement surgery. Knee 2013;20:316–18.
10. Gordon A, Kiss-Toth E, Stockley I, Eastell R, Wilkinson JM. Polymorphisms in the interleukin-1 receptor antagonist and interleukin-6 genes affect risk of osteolysis in patients with total hip arthroplasty. Arthritis Rheum 2008;58:3157–65.
11. Heuts PH, Vlaeyen JW, Roelofs J, de Bie RA, Aretz K, van Weel C, van Schayck OC. Pain-related fear and daily functioning in patients with osteoarthritis. Pain 2004;110:228–35.
12. Imamura M, Imamura ST, Kaziyama HHS, Targino RA, Hsing WT, de Souza LP, Cutait MM, Fregni F, Camanho GL. Impact of nervous system hyperalgesia on pain, disability, and quality of life in patients with knee osteoarthritis: a controlled analysis. Arthritis Rheum 2008;59:1424–31.
13. Jimenez-Andrade JM, Bloom AP, Stake JI, Mantyh WG, Taylor RN, Freeman KT, Ghilardi JR, Kuskowski MA, Mantyh PW. Pathological sprouting of adult nociceptors in chronic prostate cancer-induced bone pain. J Neurosci 2010;30:14649–56.
14. Keefe FJ, Smith SJ, Buffington AL, Gibson J, Studts JL, Caldwell DS. Recent advances and future directions in the biopsychosocial assessment and treatment of arthritis. J Consult Clin Psychol 2002;70:640.
15. Kehlet H, Jensen TS, Woolf CJ. Persistent postsurgical pain: risk factors and prevention. Lancet 2006;367:1618–25.
16. Kosek E, Ordeberg G. Abnormalities of somatosensory perception in patients with painful osteoarthritis normalize following successful treatment. Eur J Pain 2000;4:229–38.

17. Kurtz S, Ong K, Lau E, Mowat F, Helpern M. Projections of primary and revision hip and knee arthroplasty in the United States from 2005 to 2030. J Bone Joint Surg Am 2007;89:780–5.
18. Ling SM, Patel DD, Garnero P, Zhan M, Vaduganathan M, Muller D, Taub D, Bathon JM, Hochberg M, Abernethy DR, et al. Serum protein signatures detect early radiographic osteoarthritis. Osteoarthritis Cartilage 2009;17:43–8.
19. Lorig K, González VM, Laurent DD, Morgan L, Laris B. Arthritis self-management program variations: three studies. Arthritis Rheum 1998;11:448–54.
20. Lundblad H, Kreicbergs A, Jansson KA. Prediction of persistent pain after total knee replacement for osteoarthritis. J Bone Joint Surg Br 2008;90:166–71.
21. Petersen KK, Arendt-Nielsen L, Simonsen O, Wilder-Smith O, Laursen MB. Presurgical assessment of temporal summation of pain predicts the development of chronic postoperative pain 12 months after total knee replacement. Pain 2015;156:55–61.
22. Petersen KK, Simonsen O, Laursen MB, Nielsen TA, Rasmussen S, Arendt-Nielsen L. Chronic postoperative pain after primary and revision total knee arthroplasty. Clin J Pain 2015;31:1–6.
23. Phillips K, Clauw DJ. Central pain mechanisms in chronic pain states—maybe it is all in their head. Best Pract Res Clin Rheumatol 2011;25:141–54.
24. Reimann F, Cox JJ, Belfer I, Diatchenko L, Zaykin DV, McHale DP, Drenth JP, Dai F, Wheeler J, Sanders F, et al. Pain perception is altered by a nucleotide polymorphism in SCN9A. Proc Natl Acad Sci USA 2010;107:5148–53.
25. Riis A, Rathleff MS, Jensen MB, Simonsen O. Low grading of the severity of knee osteoarthritis pre-operatively is associated with a lower functional level after total knee replacement: a prospective cohort study with 12 months' follow-up. Bone Joint J 2014;96-B:1498–502.
26. Schnitzer T, Marks J. A systematic review of the efficacy and general safety of antibodies to NGF in the treatment of OA of the hip or knee. Osteoarthritis Cartilage 2015;23:S8–17.
27. Skou ST, Graven-Nielsen T, Rasmussen S, Simonsen O, Laursen MB, Arendt-Nielsen L. Widespread sensitization in patients with chronic pain after revision total knee arthroplasty. Pain 2013;154:1588–94.
28. Skou ST, Graven-Nielsen T, Rasmussen S, Simonsen O, Laursen MB, Arendt-Nielsen L. Facilitation of pain sensitization in knee osteoarthritis and persistent post-operative pain: a cross-sectional study. Eur J Pain 2014;18:1024–31.
29. Skou ST, Roos EM, Laursen MB, Rathleff MS, Arendt-Nielsen L, Simonsen O, Rasmussen S. A randomized, controlled trial of total knee replacement. N Engl J Med 2015;373:1597–606.
30. Suokas A, Walsh D, McWilliams D, Condon L, Moreton B, Wylde V, Arendt-Nielsen L, Zhang W. Quantitative sensory testing in painful osteoarthritis: a systematic review and meta-analysis. Osteoarthritis Cartilage 2012;20:1075–85.
31. Theodosiou M, Rush RA, Zhou X, Hu D, Walker J, Tracey D. Hyperalgesia due to nerve damage: role of nerve growth factor. Pain 1999;81:245–55.
32. Wilder-Smith OH, Schreyer T, Scheffer GJ, Arendt-Nielsen L. Patients with chronic pain after abdominal surgery show less preoperative endogenous pain

inhibition and more postoperative hyperalgesia: a pilot study. J Pain Palliat Care Pharmacother 2010;24:119–28.

33. Wylde V, Sayers A, Lenguerrand E, Gooberman-Hill R, Pyke M, Beswick AD, Dieppe P, Blom AW. Preoperative widespread pain sensitization and chronic pain after hip and knee replacement: a cohort analysis. Pain 2015;156:47.
34. Yarnitsky D, Crispel Y, Eisenberg E, Granovsky Y, Ben-Nun A, Sprecher E, Best LA, Granot M. Prediction of chronic post-operative pain: pre-operative DNIC testing identifies patients at risk. Pain 2008;138:22–8.
35. Yusuf E, Kortekaas MC, Watt I, Huizinga TW, Kloppenburg M. Do knee abnormalities visualised on MRI explain knee pain in knee osteoarthritis? A systematic review. Ann Rheum Dis 2011;70:60–7.

CHAPTER 12

# New Treatment Opportunities

*David A. Walsh*

Musculoskeletal pain remains an increasing source of distress and disability for the world's aging population. Osteoarthritis (OA) is the commonest form of arthritis, and low back pain remains the greatest musculoskeletal source of disability in people of working age. Pain perceived as originating from the joint in rheumatoid arthritis (RA) or fibromyalgia (FM) represents diverse contributions from peripheral and central mechanisms. Arthritis pain results from complex interactions between joint pathology, neuronal processing, and psychological context. Current treatments might offer only partial relief, and combination approaches are often necessary. This complexity challenges both patients and health professionals, but also provides opportunities for new treatments and to better harness the benefits of existing treatments.

## CURRENT TREATMENT GUIDELINES

Published guidelines and reviews summarize current evidence of benefits for a range of treatments [4, 10, 15, 18], although many people use few, or sometimes none. Active patient participation should be encouraged, with exercise, systemic analgesic drugs, psychological approaches, and multidisciplinary therapies, each offering benefit to people with OA, RA, low back pain, or FM. People with OA or RA might additionally benefit from orthotic devices, locally administered drugs, or joint replacement surgery, and those with low back pain from manipulation/mobilization, from radiofrequency nerve ablation or surgical fusion. Many more treatments have displayed less certain efficacy in randomized controlled trials (RCTs). Effect sizes are often small compared with placebos, and trial durations are often shorter than musculoskeletal pain's often protracted time course. RCTs might lack statistical power needed to detect important adverse events.

Acetaminophen (paracetamol) has received little scrutiny in RCTs despite its widespread use. Nonsteroidal anti-inflammatory drugs (NSAIDs) might be of benefit for OA, RA, or low back pain, and opioids might help OA, but tolerance, adverse events, and dependency might limit their use. Newer opioids with mixed modes of action have shown some positive effects. Tricyclic antidepressants or gabapentinoids might improve pain in FM [4], although evidence for OA, RA, and low back pain is less convincing. Serotonin norepinephrine reuptake inhibitors (SNRIs) such as duloxetine or milnacipran display small incremental benefits over placebo in reducing pain from OA or FM. Local glucocorticosteroid injections relieve pain in OA and RA, but benefits above placebos in low back pain are typically small and short lived. Topical NSAIDs or capsaicin might relieve hand or knee pain associated with OA, and might cause fewer serious adverse events than do oral NSAIDs.

## TREATMENT UPTAKE AND STRATIFICATION

The heterogeneous experience of joint pain reflects multiple mechanisms, and no treatment will be effective for all symptoms in everyone. Joint pains might be attributed different qualities, such as aching or burning, dull or sharp, some overlapping with inflammatory pain, or neuropathic pain. Joint pain might be intermittent and precipitated or exacerbated by mechanical factors. It is sometimes continuous and often spontaneous. Patients might try out many interventions before they eventually find those that most effectively relieve their pain. Each treatment poses its own risk, and failing treatment encourages disengagement while still risking adverse events. Facilitating early access and adherence to those interventions that will be most effective for the individual could improve patient outcomes from existing therapies.

Treatment uptake and continued use depend not only on pain severity, but also on patients' beliefs, convenience, cost, and other social factors [14]. Believing that OA is an inevitable part of older age about which nothing can be done and negative attitudes from the general practitioner each contributes to lower primary care consultation. Different people evaluate benefits and risks from treatment differently, varying in their willingness to accept risks of serious medical events such as heart attack, stroke, or stomach bleed [13].

Selecting treatments that are matched to underlying pain mechanisms is supported by an important, albeit limited, evidence base. Glucocorticoid injections might be most effective for people with RA, or for some with OA. However, ultrasound evidence of synovitis has not reliably identified those people with knee OA who would gain benefit from injection [6]. Components of synovitis that mediate pain and are responsive to glucocorticoid might not be those that are observed by ultrasound. Placebo effects might not be specific to inflammatory pain mechanisms. Nerve growth factor (NGF) blockade reduces peripheral sensitization, and might be more effective for OA than for neuropathic pain, whereas pregabalin acts on central pain mechanisms and might be more effective in neuropathic pain or FM than in OA.

A patient's understanding of his or her joint pain might differ substantially from the mechanistic basis underpinning the therapist's approach. Psychological interventions might be resisted if they seem to invalidate the patient's problem. Understanding and acknowledging the patient's prior experience and perspective, and combining effective educational tools and risk assessment with ongoing interpretation of benefits and harm during treatment exposure are key factors when maximizing benefit from any treatment. Patients (and physicians) might be reluctant to use analgesics to mask pain, and people are unlikely to exercise if they believe that doing this will exacerbate joint damage. Such beliefs are reinforced by temporary increases in pain during exercise and, sometimes accidentally, by diagnostic explanations such as wear and tear or degenerative. Continued activity and exercise are beneficial for most forms of chronic musculoskeletal pain, and normal activities do not typically damage joints. Fear avoidance for activity can contribute to disability, and can be reduced by cognitive behavioral approaches. Fear of treatment can be a barrier to effective pain management.

Treatments might be cost-effective only for selected patient subgroups that are concealed within negative RCTs. Patient stratification might improve treatment outcomes for low back pain [5]. Criteria for subgrouping people with OA or FM require robust evaluation prior to their widespread implementation. People with unfavorable prognosis have most to gain from treatment, especially those treatments directed to modifiable risk factors. Neuropathy or central pain augmentation might predominate only in a proportion of people with OA, and improved pain phenotyping might define patient groups for whom existing treatments would have greater benefit. Early treatment discontinuation in nonresponders reduces unnecessary risk of adverse events. High body mass index or low mood might significantly predict worse than average outcomes from arthroplasty, but those outcomes might still be worthwhile. It is currently uncertain whether presurgical weight reduction strategies or psychological interventions provide clinically important benefits.

## NEW PHARMACOLOGICAL TARGETS

Novel pharmacological targets are being identified through increased understanding of joint pain mechanisms. Drugs that have been developed for other indications are being repurposed to the potential benefit of people with arthritis. Treatments that target underlying disease mechanisms should also reduce pain, as demonstrated both for traditional and biologic disease-modifying agents in RA. However, even in RA, pain remains the most important problem for many patients, and amelioration of pain can be incomplete, despite remission of inflammatory disease. In conditions such as OA, back pain, and FM, fundamental disease mechanisms are incompletely understood, and the Holy Grail of disease modification has yet to be attained. The often weak associations between pain and imaged joint structure in OA and back pain reflect discrepancies between those pathological features that permit diagnostic classification and those that mediate pain. Structural pain modification should aim to permanently relieve or prevent progression of symptoms, rather than necessarily to preserve normal appearances of the joint.

Pharmacological interventions aim to reduce joint pathology, to directly modify peripheral or central nerve function, or to optimize endogenous central pain modulation. Within the joint, synovial inflammation can contribute to pain. Targeting peripheral mechanisms might not only relieve pain, but also retard structural damage. Attempts at OA disease modification by slowing progression of joint-space narrowing on plain radiographs have been largely unsuccessful and occasionally associated with increased pain [9]. Structural changes that might contribute more to OA pain than does joint-space narrowing include loss of osteochondral integrity associated with full-thickness cartilage defects and osteochondral angiogenesis, and neoinnervation of structures that are not normally supplied by sensory nerves, such as the noncalcified articular cartilage and the inner two-thirds of knee menisci. Sensory nerves might be exposed to biomechanical or chemical stimulation, leading to direct neuronal activation or to increased sensitization. Changes in central sensitization might be driven by ongoing nociceptive transmission, and also augmented by local or systemic factors related to genetic background, comorbidities, inflammation, and neuropsychological processes, including mood and sleep disturbance.

The synovial joint provides an ideal compartment for local drug administration, either topically or by intra-articular injection. Analgesic benefits of glucocorticoid injections in knee OA, for example, can be prolonged, and topical NSAIDs can offer useful relief of hand or knee OA pain. Drugs with pharmacokinetic or physical properties that preclude systemic administration might yet be appropriate for local injection [12], and drugs with poor penetration to the central nervous system (e.g., monoclonal antibodies) might avoid adverse events such as somnolence and nausea. However, substance injected into the synovial cavity might not access all relevant joint compartments. Subchondral bone might be separated from the synovial cavity by an impermeable osteochondral junction, at least in early OA. For some people, central mechanisms might predominate, for example, in FM, where peripherally acting anti-inflammatory agents have little evidence of benefit. Local treatments might alter central pain mechanisms by removing the drive to central sensitization, or directly through placebo effects.

## Inflammation

In RA, biologic agents that specifically target tumor necrosis factor alpha (TNF-α), IL-1, IL-6, or B cells each improves pain in people with active inflammatory disease, and traditional disease-modifying antirheumatic drugs similarly improve both inflammation and pain in RA [18]. Synovitis contributes to joint pain also in OA. Cyclooxygenase inhibitors, administered locally or systemically, and local glucocorticoid injections each relieves OA pain. However, TNF-α-blocking antibodies have little analgesic benefit in OA [1], possibly indicating that different mediators might drive inflammatory pain in OA and RA. RCTs are ongoing in OA of hydroxychloroquine, another drug that has been found helpful in RA [7].

Inflammation might facilitate pain not only by activating joint nociceptors, but also by driving changes in peripheral and central pain processing. Systemic inflammation might also mediate associations between musculoskeletal pain and high body mass index, metabolic syndrome, or other comorbidities. Targeting neuroimmune interactions, microglia, astrocytes, and their products with drugs that cross the blood–brain barrier might reduce central sensitization.

## Subchondral Bone Turnover

Subchondral bone marrow lesions (BMLs) detected by magnetic resonance imaging (MRI) are associated with OA pain both in cross-sectional and prospective studies, and also might precede worsening cartilage loss. BMLs are associated with increased bone turnover, and increased subchondral osteoclast activity characterizes OA both in human and in other animals. Reducing osteoclast activation can relieve OA pain and might retard structural damage. The bisphosphonate zoledronic acid reduced pain behavior and structural damage in rat OA models, and a pilot RCT indicated reduced pain and BMLs in people with OA, following a single zoledronate infusion [8]. Confirmation in an ongoing definitive RCT is eagerly awaited. Similarly, osteoprotegerin and cathepsin K inhibitors both inhibited subchondral osteoclast activity and reduced pain behavior or electrophysiological evidence of sensitization in preclinical models. The extent of analgesia observed with these agents is disproportionate to reductions in cartilage damage or osteophytosis, suggesting that osteoclast activation might be more important for pain than are traditional structural parameters.

## Mechanotransduction

Intermittent pain experienced during joint movement or loading emphasizes the biomechanical component of joint pain. Normal biomechanical stimulation can initiate pain in the presence of neuronal sensitization. Intermittent joint pain is often so severe that it prevents normal activity, and is resistant to traditional analgesics except in doses that incur intolerable adverse events. Inhibiting mechanotransduction should relieve musculoskeletal pain. Corrections of biomechanical abnormalities by exercise, orthotic, or surgical approaches continue to be a cornerstone of modern treatment. Mechanotransduction also depends on the localization of sensory nerve terminals within the joint, on specific mechanosensitive ion channels, and on interactions between nerves and their cellular and matrix environments [19]. Mechanosensitive nerves are normally inhibited by specific cell matrix interactions, and their increased activity in arthritis might be caused not only by increased expression or phosphorylation, but also by release from normal suppression. Mechanotransduction is also essential for non-nociceptive physiology, including hearing and cardiovascular regulation, but nociception-specific pathways offer hope as novel analgesic targets.

## Peripheral Sensitization

Analgesic benefits in recent clinical trials of NGF-blocking antibodies [16] support the proposed importance of peripheral sensitization in

OA pain. Several clinical development programs recommenced following release of Food and Drug Administration hold on clinical trials involving NGF-blocking antibodies in early 2015. In parallel, tyrosine kinase inhibitors have been developed that block the TrkA receptor for NGF. Possible off-target effects due to limited selectivity have been partially circumvented by localized intra-articular delivery [12], or development of allosteric inhibitors selective for TrkA compared with TrkB, TrkC, and other tyrosine kinases [11]. Evidence from preclinical OA models supports analgesic efficacy comparable to NGF-blocking antibodies. However, incomplete understanding of the rare adverse event of rapidly progressive OA that has been observed with NGF-blocking antibodies advises a cautious and comprehensive assessment of potential toxicity. Calcitonin gene-related peptide (CGRP)–blocking antibodies might also reduce peripheral sensitization and are showing promising signs in clinical trials for migraine. However, a RCT of LY2951742 compared with placebo or celecoxib for OA pain was terminated following interim analysis in 2015 because of lack of efficacy of the CGRP-blocking antibody, despite expected benefits from celecoxib [3]. Further analysis of these trial data might yet identify responsive subgroups of people with OA who have CGRP-mediated pain augmentation.

## Central Sensitization

The important contributions of central sensitization to chronic musculoskeletal pain are increasingly recognized, although their precise biomolecular and cellular mechanisms, and clinical correlates remain incompletely understood. Spinal pain pathways change during the development of experimental arthritis, amplifying nociceptive signals from the joint. Concurrently, interactions between emotional, cognitive, and sensory pathways within the brain not only exacerbate the pain experience, but also modulate descending facilitatory or inhibitory influences on spinal pain transmission. The neuropathic-like qualities of some FM and OA pain might indicate shared mechanisms between musculoskeletal and neuropathic pain. Nerve damage might follow joint surgery, explaining some persistent pain after knee arthroplasty, although neuropathology, as opposed to neuroplasticity, has not consistently been demonstrated during the progression of arthritis.

Treatments recommended for neuropathic pain, including tricyclic antidepressants, gabapentinoids, or SNRIs, might also be helpful for musculoskeletal pain conditions such as FM that are associated with central sensitization. Augmented central pain processing is also recognized in OA and RA, but might predominate in only a minority of patients. RCTs have revealed some weak evidence of benefit from antineuropathic treatments for OA pain [2]. Heterogeneity within unselected patient groups might conceal greater benefit for subgroups in whom central mechanisms play a greater contribution to their pain. Ongoing clinical trials focus on patient subgroups with high scores on neuropathic pain questionnaires. Associations between pain and mood or sleep disturbance and fatigue might be mediated by common central mechanisms, and treatments that target shared mechanisms might have greater impact on quality of life. However, mechanisms underlying these associations remain incompletely understood, and combination approaches are currently necessary to address multiple symptoms.

## PHYSICAL TREATMENTS

Exercise-based treatments remain the cornerstone of management for most musculoskeletal pain conditions. Pain impacts on quality of life not only as a symptom in its own right, but also by preventing engagement in valued activities. Exercise might directly lead to improvements in pain by altering joint biomechanics, facilitating endogenous analgesic pathways, and by suppressing pain augmentation, and indirectly might reduce the impact of pain by increasing physical and aerobic capacity and improving psychological well-being.

Physical treatments might fall under several categories, including manipulation/mobilization, strengthening, stretching or mobility exercises directed at specific joint regions, treatments aiming to improve general aerobic fitness and function, and behavioral interventions targeting posture, gait, kinesiophobia, or activity cycling. Physical treatments are underpinned by a range of hypothesized pain mechanisms, although head-to-head RCTs have often not demonstrated clear superiority of one approach over another. For example, in low back pain, similar benefits have been observed across a range of manipulation/mobilization, strengthening/stretching/postural, and general aerobic approaches. Modern physiotherapy practice often employs a combination of approaches personalized to individual needs and response.

## PSYCHOLOGICAL INTERVENTIONS

Emotional factors are key components of the pain experience, and improving psychological outcomes is an essential attribute of interventions that treat chronic pain. Psychological factors might not only influence the emotional response and impact of pain, but, through linked neuronal pathways within the brain, also drive sensitization and descending pain modulation. Adverse psychological factors such as anxiety and low mood predict musculoskeletal pain onset and worse pain outcomes across low back pain, OA, RA, and FM. Psychological factors also predict responses to a range of treatment modalities, ranging from usual conservative care through surgical procedures. Psychological interventions, therefore, have the potential not only to ameliorate pain's emotional components and improve coping, but also to remove barriers to recovery, to improve utilization and facilitate response to other treatments, and to directly modify the sensory component of pain.

Cognitive behavioral therapy (CBT) might be helpful in OA, low back pain, or FM, although, as patient and professional beliefs vary between diagnoses, specific content of cognitive interventions should be adapted to the individual. Fear of pain and fear of activities that might induce at least short-term symptom exacerbation are common across all these conditions, although fear of injury or damage might be particularly associated with diagnoses attributed to biomechanical causes such as OA and low back pain. Low intensity or short-duration CBT might usefully reduce fear of pain or activity in FM and facilitate recovery in low back pain in appropriately selected patients. Other psychological approaches show promise for improving joint pain and its impact, either alone or as adjuncts to CBT. Motivational interviewing has demonstrated benefit in FM, where high levels of fatigue might particularly impact on engagement in active treatments [4]. Acceptance and Commitment Therapy and mindfulness approaches focus on pursing life values, despite the presence of pain, rather than pursuing goals that might never be achieved.

## COMBINATION TREATMENTS

Combination therapies are attractive when several treatment modalities display evidence of benefit, but no single treatment alone can cure joint pain. Targeting different mechanisms at different points on the pain pathway might be more effective than acting on a single mechanism. Changes to health care provision might be required to permit coordinated provision of medical, physical, and psychological interventions. Empirical evidence is required to inform combination therapy, but clinical trials for complex interventions are expensive and difficult to undertake. Combinations might be most successful when there is treatment synergy or where interventions address different patient outcomes, although incremental benefit from each additional therapeutic component might still be small. Combination therapy is often tested as a care package, for example, a multidisciplinary pain management program, recognizing interdependence between physical, psychological, and medical components. Specific benefits from each component of these packages cannot be fully defined. Different approaches might achieve similar outcomes. Acceptability, availability, converging beliefs between patients and therapists, and compatibility with concurrent treatments might be more important than specific content in determining clinical benefit.

Combination therapies run the risk of increased or unexpected toxicity. Rapidly progressive OA following exposure to NGF-blocking antibodies was associated in retrospective analyses with concomitant NSAID use. Interactions with over-the-counter preparations raise particular regulatory concerns when it might be difficult to ensure that patients are fully informed of potential risks.

Combination of weight reduction strategies with psychological or physiotherapeutic interventions might further improve OA knee pain [17], thereby improving functional and psychological outcomes. CBT alone might have rather modest long-term benefits in FM or low back pain, although CBT approaches can augment responses to physiotherapy. Psychological approaches that address fear of activity or low motivation might facilitate adherence to exercise recommendations [4]. Multidisciplinary approaches typically address multiple problems concurrently, including not only pain, but also fatigue, mood disturbance, and disability.

## CONCLUSIONS

The management of joint pain has undergone step changes in recent years. The theoretical framework for arthritis pain has shifted from a unique focus on joint damage and inflammation to a more sophisticated understanding of the interplay between central and peripheral mechanisms. Treatments that target the joint remain key to improving patient outcomes, but cannot alone provide satisfactory relief for all patients. Treatments acting on central pain mechanisms are moving from centrally acting analgesics such as opiates that might suppress any pain, but are associated with important adverse events, to selectively targeting mechanisms at key points in pain pathways. Increased understanding of the links between pain experience and pain mechanism is leading to interventions that target key aspects of pain, more sophisticated evaluation of those aspects of pain that display clinically important improvement in response to specific treatments, and targeting of treatments to those people who are most likely to benefit from them. This multimodal approach to pain management raises important questions about the benefits and risks of treatment combinations compared with monotherapies. In some respects, all analgesic interventions are complex, and response depends on the context in which they are delivered [20]. Genetic constitution, comorbidities, specific joint pathology, plasticity within the nervous system, and psychological and social factors each contribute to pain and treatment response. Improving how we deliver treatments for arthritis pain offers great hope for better relief of suffering in the years to come.

## ACKNOWLEDGMENTS

The author declares no financial support for the preparation of this article. He has provided paid consultancy during 2015 to Novartis Consumer Health SA, a GSK Consumer Healthcare company and is principle investigator on an investigator-led research grant funded by Pfizer Ltd. Neither commercial entity has contributed to the preparation of this manuscript.

## REFERENCES

1. Chevalier X, Ravaud P, Maheu E, Baron G, Rialland A, Vergnaud P, Roux C, Maugars Y, Mulleman D, Lukas C, et al. Adalimumab in patients with hand osteoarthritis refractory to analgesics and NSAIDs: a randomised, multicentre, double-blind, placebo-controlled trial. Ann Rheum Dis 2015;74:1697–705.
2. Citrome L, Weiss-Citrome A. A systematic review of duloxetine for osteoarthritic pain: what is the number needed to treat, number needed to harm, and likelihood to be helped or harmed? Postgrad Med 2012;124:83–93.
3. Ely Lilly and Company. A study of LY2951742 in participants with mild to moderate osteoarthritis knee pain 2015 [cited November 21, 2015]. Accessed at https://clinicaltrials.gov/ct2/show/NCT02192190.
4. Fitzcharles MA, Ste-Marie PA, Goldenberg DL, Pereira JX, Abbey S, Choiniere M, Ko G, Moulin DE, Panopalis P, Proulx J, et al. 2012 Canadian Guidelines for the diagnosis and management of fibromyalgia syndrome: executive summary. Pain Res Manag 2013;18:119–26.
5. Hill JC, Whitehurst DG, Lewis M, Bryan S, Dunn KM, Foster NE, Konstantinou K, Main CJ, Mason E, Somerville S, et al. Comparison of stratified primary care management for low back pain with current best practice (STarT Back): a randomised controlled trial. Lancet 2011;378:1560–71.
6. Hirsch G, Kitas G, Klocke R. Intra-articular corticosteroid injection in osteoarthritis of the knee and hip: factors predicting pain relief: a systematic review. Semin Arthritis Rheum 2013;42:451–73.
7. Kingsbury SR, Tharmanathan P, Adamson J, Arden NK, Birrell F, Cockayne S, Dickson J, Doherty M, Dziedzic KS, Grainger A, et al. Hydroxychloroquine

effectiveness in reducing symptoms of hand osteoarthritis (HERO): study protocol for a randomized controlled trial. Trials 2013;14:64.
8. Laslett LL, Dore DA, Quinn SJ, Boon P, Ryan E, Winzenberg TM, Jones G. Zoledronic acid reduces knee pain and bone marrow lesions over 1 year: a randomised controlled trial. Ann Rheum Dis 2012;71:1322–8.
9. Lohmander LS, Hellot S, Dreher D, Krantz EF, Kruger DS, Guermazi A, Eckstein F. Intraarticular sprifermin (recombinant human fibroblast growth factor 18) in knee osteoarthritis: a randomized, double-blind, placebo-controlled trial. Arthritis Rheum 2014;66:1820–31.
10. McAlindon TE, Bannuru RR, Sullivan MC, Arden NK, Berenbaum F, Bierma-Zeinstra SM, Hawker GA, Henrotin Y, Hunter DJ, Kawaguchi H, et al. OARSI guidelines for the non-surgical management of knee osteoarthritis. Osteoarthritis Cartilage 2014;22:363–88.
11. Nwosu LN, Mapp PI, Chapman V, Walsh DA. Blocking the tropomyosin receptor kinase A (TrkA) receptor inhibits pain behaviour in two rat models of osteoarthritis. Ann Rheum Dis. doi:10.1136/annrheumdis-2014-207203.
12. ONO Pharmaceutical Co. Ltd. A study to evaluate safety, tolerability, pharmacokinetics and pharmacology of ONO-4474 in healthy volunteers 2015 [cited October 21, 2015]. Accessed at https://clinicaltrials.gov/ct2/show/NCT02454387.
13. Richardson CG, Chalmers A, Llewellyn-Thomas HA, Klinkhoff A, Carswell A, Kopec JA. Pain relief in osteoarthritis: patients' willingness to risk medication-induced gastrointestinal, cardiovascular, and cerebrovascular complications. J Rheumatol 2007;34:1569–75.
14. Rosemann T, Joos S, Szecsenyi J, Laux G, Wensing M. Health service utilization patterns of primary care patients with osteoarthritis. BMC Health Serv Res 2007;7:169.
15. Savigny P, Watson P, Underwood M, Guideline Development Group. Early management of persistent non-specific low back pain: summary of NICE guidance. BMJ 2009;338:b1805.
16. Schnitzer TJ, Marks JA. A systematic review of the efficacy and general safety of antibodies to NGF in the treatment of OA of the hip or knee. Osteoarthritis Cartilage 2015;23:S8–17.
17. Somers TJ, Blumenthal JA, Guilak F, Kraus VB, Schmitt DO, Babyak MA, Craighead LW, Caldwell DS, Rice JR, McKee DC, et al. Pain coping skills training and lifestyle behavioral weight management in patients with knee osteoarthritis: a randomized controlled study. Pain 2012;153:1199–209.
18. Walsh DA, McWilliams DF. Mechanisms, impact and management of pain in rheumatoid arthritis. Nat Rev Rheumatol 2014;10:581–92.
19. Wood JN, Eijkelkamp N. Noxious mechanosensation: molecules and circuits. Curr Opin Pharmacol 2012;12:4–8.
20. Zhang W, Robertson J, Jones AC, Dieppe PA, Doherty M. The placebo effect and its determinants in osteoarthritis: meta-analysis of randomised controlled trials. Ann Rheumat Dis 2008;67:1716–23.

CHAPTER 13

# Alternative Treatment Options for Osteoarthritis—Glucosamine and Chondroitin: Facts and Evidence

*Stephan Reichenbach*

Osteoarthritis is the most common joint disorder. It is a form of arthritis that causes pathological changes to the whole joint, including cartilage, bones, synovia, and muscles. Hands, knees, and hips are common sites of osteoarthritis. Patients may suffer joint pain or stiffness or complain about lost function [3, 7]. Osteoarthritis is a debilitating and painful disease that reduces quality of life for millions of people around the world.

Although prevalence rates are hard to establish because definitions differ, population studies that measured osteoarthritis prevalence with radiographs in the United States and Europe suggest that about 24% of those above 45 and about 44% of those above 80 have knee osteoarthritis. A Dutch study found that knee osteoarthritis symptoms were present in about 12–15% of those 55 and older. Since osteoarthritis tends to worsen over time, and there is, as yet, no proven therapy that repairs the underlying structural damage to cartilage, patients who are not yet symptomatic may develop them later [3, 7]. As the population ages, osteoarthritis will grow more prevalent, further burdening the health care system.

## GLUCOSAMINE AND CHONDROITIN

Because there is still no evidence-based treatment to halt or roll back the progress of the disease, physicians and patients usually focus on reducing osteoarthritis symptoms. Doctors often prescribe analgesics and nonsteroidal anti-inflammatory drugs to treat pain and to increase mobility, but these drugs can have serious gastrointestinal and cardiovascular side effects [17, 20]. Since no treatments dependably cure the underlying problems of osteoarthritis, patients and doctors may turn to supplements that promise relief. All parties would welcome a method that preserves existing cartilage or help it grow back, and some manufacturers market the food supplements glucosamine and chondroitin to patients with osteoarthritis, claiming that these supplements will help stabilize or regrow joint cartilage and reduce pain. In Europe and Asia, these supplements are available by prescription, and can be bought over the counter in the United States and Australia [8].

Glucosamine is an amino sugar in bones, fungi, and shells. It is a building block for part of the structure of cartilage called glycosaminoglycans. Glucosamine usually comes in pill form, and sometimes as an injection. It may be taken alone, as glucosamine hydrochloride or sulfate, or combined with other supplements, such as chondroitin. Chondroitin is a highly hydrophilic, gel-forming polysaccharide macromolecule that enables cartilage to resist compression, usually extracted from cow, pig, or shark cartilage and taken in the form of chondroitin sulfate [13]. In 2008, in the United States, adults used more glucosamine than any other nonmineral supplement [1].

## STUDY RESULTS

Randomized trials to test the efficacy of glucosamine and chondroitin have produced conflicting results, which range from showing significant beneficial effects [5] to showing no effect at all [4]. Results of the first systematic reviews and meta-analyses on glucosamine and chondroitin use were also conflicting [22]. While scientists view inconclusive results with caution, supplement markets thrive on them, publicizing positive studies and ignoring those with negative results. For example, many websites that sell these supplements list randomized controlled trials (RCTs) and meta-analyses that seem to support their claims.

In 2000, McAlindon et al. [11] published an influential systematic quality assessment and meta-analysis of the efficacy of glucosamine and chondroitin in JAMA. Although McAlindon's team found that studies showed these supplements had moderate-to-large beneficial effect, they urged their results be interpreted with caution, since most included studies were poor quality or were supported by a manufacturer. Overall, there was indication of publication bias. When McAlindon et al. [11] considered only high-quality and large trials, benefit diminished. Richey et al. [14] offered no such cautions in their 2003 meta-analysis of 15 studies published or performed between 1980 and 2002. When they assessed the effectiveness of oral glucosamine or chondroitin for knee or hip osteoarthritis, they described the trials as homogenous and unequivocally endorsed their positive results.

In 2005, Towheed et al. [19] wrote the first *Cochrane Review* of glucosamine therapy for osteoarthritis. Their study analyzed 20 RCTs and found that glucosamine significantly reduced joint pain. But, when they limited their analysis to the eight studies that were adequately concealed, glucosamine no longer provided the benefit of reducing pain. That same year, McAlindon and Biggee [10] questioned the effectiveness of glucosamine and chondroitin, based on null results of clinical trials not funded by industry. When Towheed et al.'s [19] review was updated in 2009 to include 25 RCTs, results were similar.

Large, high-quality RCTs were in short supply until 2006, when the results of the U.S. National Center for Complementary and Integrative Health GAIT Study were published in the *New England Journal of Medicine* [4]. The trial was high quality, large (1583 patients), randomized, and placebo controlled. It sought to determine whether glucosamine and/or chondroitin reduced pain from knee osteoarthritis. The 4-year study, carried out at 16 sites, showed that, overall, the supplements (alone or together) did not significantly relieve pain. However, one of several subgroup analyses suggested that patients whose knee pain was moderate to severe might benefit from the combined therapy [4].

A trend over time soon became apparent: The appearance of more large, high-quality RCTs began to shift the results of glucosamine and chondroitin studies from significantly positive to generally null.

In 2007, Reichenbach et al. [13] published a systematic review and meta-analysis of available RCTs to see whether chondroitin affected pain and to find out whether the beneficial effects reported in RCTs could be explained by biases within individual trials or publication bias. The 20 trials we considered had allocated a total of 4056 patients, mostly with knee osteoarthritis, to chondroitin, placebo, or a nonintervention control group. Although all but one of these trials reported that it had been randomized, only one trial had an adequately generated allocation sequence, and only two trials adequately concealed allocation. Only three trials had a placebo control group, and only three analyzed based on intention-to-treat. It was unclear how missing data were dealt with in most trials, and eight trials imputed by carrying forward the last observation. More recent trials were usually bigger than earlier trials and were better constructed. The percentage of patients with low-grade osteoarthritis was also lower in more recent trials [13].

Reichenbach et al. [13] found that the effect size of chondroitin was large (−0.75; 95% confidence interval [CI], −0.99 to −0.50), but only if they included all trials. Because the trials were heterogeneous, it was hard to interpret their results. Three methodological characteristics appeared to account for heterogeneity: concealing allocation, intention-to-treat analysis, and sample size. When poor quality trials were included in the meta-analysis, this inflated the benefits of chondroitin and increased between-trial heterogeneity. But, when only the trials with large samples and an intention-to-treat analysis were included (accounting for 40% of randomly assigned patients), effect size dropped to almost 0. There was no clinically relevant benefit of chondroitin. In addition, newer publications showed smaller effects than older publications, and the benefits of chondroitin decreased by an effect size of 0.08 per year (CI, 0.04–0.12; $P < 0.001$). Finally, trials in which experimental and control groups used similar analgesic co-interventions showed less benefit than trials in which controls used more analgesics or trials that provided no information on analgesic use. Effect size was not associated with follow-up duration, maximum length of treatment, or chondroitin dosage [13].

Reichenbach et al. [13] pointed out that their results and McAlindon's are not contradictory. Instead, they show a trend over time: As higher-quality evidence has accumulated, effect sizes have decreased. Reichenbach's group also took a more conservative approach to calculating effect sizes, using pooled SD to divide differences between groups instead of using SD in the control group. Reichenbach et al. also noted that higher-quality, more recent trials have a smaller proportion of patients with low-grade osteoarthritis and that it is possible this group might benefit from treatment with chondroitin: A high-quality trial that includes only patients with low-grade osteoarthritis could be conducted to answer this question.

Also in 2007, Vlad et al. [21] analyzed 15 trials that compared glucosamine with placebo, and found the pooled effect size was –0.35 (95% CI, –0.56 to –0.14) for glucosamine, again noting that studies were heterogeneous. The only feature of study design that seemed to explain this heterogeneity was concealment of allocation. When Vlad et al. [21] limited their analysis to trials that adequately concealed allocation, trials not sponsored by industry, and trials that evaluated glucosamine hydrochloride, they found glucosamine had less beneficial effects. Like earlier researchers [2], they found that trials with industry involvement showed consistently higher effect size. Vlad et al. [21] concluded that glucosamine hydrochloride was not effective but admitted it was possible that glucosamine sulfate could have a clinically relevant effect. The ancillary glucosamine/chondroitin arthritis intervention trial (GAIT) study results were issued in 2008 [15]. This double-blind, 24-month, placebo-controlled study included 572 participants from the 2006 GAIT study, and again found that the difference between treatment groups was not statistically significant, though there was a trend to improvement in patients with Stage 2 osteoarthritis. When Sawitzke et al. [16] published the 2-year GAIT study results in mid-2010, the results were much the same. The supplements had no significant benefit in reducing pain or increasing function, but there was an insignificant beneficial trend for those who took glucosamine. The GAIT study and others convinced the Osteoarthritis Research Society International

(OARSI) that evidence for the effectiveness of glucosamine sulfate and chondroitin was thinner than they had originally believed and that the supplements had no significant effect, which changed their recommendations for osteoarthritis treatment guidelines [23, 24].

In 2010, Wandel et al. [22] performed a Bayesian network meta-analysis on the effects of glucosamine, chondroitin, or placebo on patients with hip or knee osteoarthritis. The study measured the outcomes of absolute pain intensity and change in joint space width. Unlike earlier meta-analysis, Wandel et al. [22] did include the GAIT trial and limited included trials to those that averaged at least 100 patients with knee or hip osteoarthritis per arm, to avoid small sample bias [12]. A notable difference between the analysis of Wandel et al. [22] and the earlier studies by Vlad et al. [21] and Reichenbach et al. [13] is that Wandel's group chose a technique that allowed them to analyze data recorded at different time points in the RCTs and compared glucosamine and chondroitin with placebo, and with each other. They chose this method to address earlier concerns about time dependency of effects, quality control of preparations, and differences between formulations of glucosamine. The Wandel study included in its network meta-analysis 12 reports describing 10 trials. The combined trials had randomly allocated 3803 patients to one or the other experimental interventions or placebo. Six trials adequately concealed allocation, and nine blinded patients adequately. Seven trials performed an intention-to-treat analysis. Supplement manufacturers funded all but three trials. Eight trials instituted quality controls to ensure adequate concentrations of glucosamine and chondroitin. Overall difference in pain intensity versus placebo, based on a summary of all time points, was −0.4 cm (95% credible interval, −0.7 to −0.1 cm) on a 10-cm visual analog scale for glucosamine, −0.3 cm (−0.7 to 0.0 cm) for chondroitin, and −0.5 cm (−0.9 to 0.0 cm) for the combination of glucosamine and chondroitin. Corresponding effect sizes were −0.17 (−0.28 to −0.05) for glucosamine, −0.13 (−0.27 to 0.00) for chondroitin, and −0.19 (−0.37 to 0.00) for the combination (Fig. 13-1) [22].

Wandel et al. [22] concluded that there was no evidence for time-dependent effects and that poor quality control did not account for the failure of glucosamine and chondroitin supplements to produce

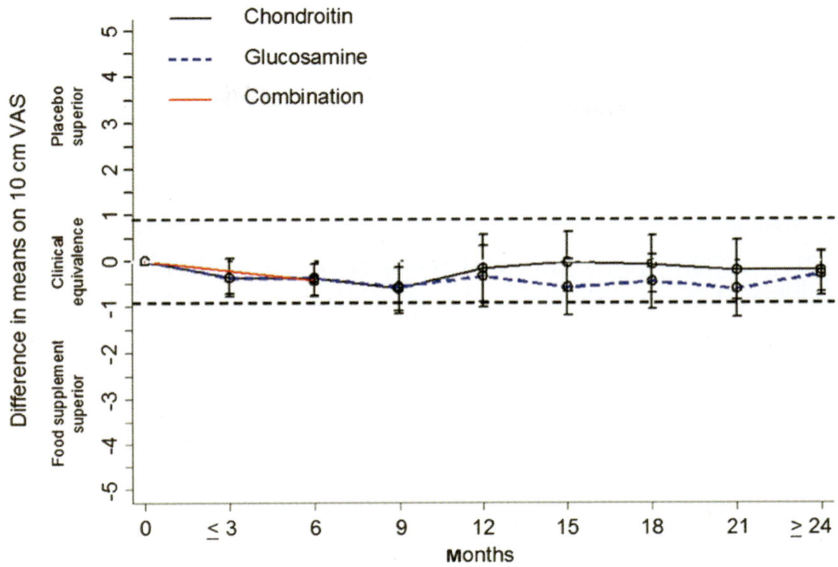


**FIGURE 13-1** Differences in pain intensity measured on visual analog scale (VAS) between experimental interventions and placebo over time. The darker shading between −0.9 and +0.9 cm represents area of clinical equivalence. Negative values indicate benefit of experimental interventions compared with placebo. Pain reductions of −0.9 cm or more are deemed clinically relevant, smaller differences are not. (Adapted from Wandel et al. [22].)

clinically relevant effects. Wandel et al.'s [22] network meta-analysis showed that neither chondroitin nor glucosamine, nor their combination, had any clinically relevant effect on the amount of joint pain patients felt. They also found that glucosamine sulfate had no clinically relevant effect.

In a 2015 paper that detailed an Australian industry-independent, large, double-blind, randomized, placebo-controlled clinical trial long-term evaluation of glucosamine sulfate study (LEGS) with 2-year follow-up, Fransen et al. [8] affirmed that glucosamine and chondroitin provide no significant symptom relief. This study evaluated the separate and combined effect of glucosamine and chondroitin on joint pain. Glucosamine or chondroitin treatment did not reduce knee pain, whether taken alone or in combination.

Glucosamine, chondroitin, and their combination are no better than placebo at reducing joint pain. Treatment benefits, where they appear to exist, may be overestimated because of methodological shortcomings, small sample bias, or industry influence. Insurers and health authorities should not pay for these preparations [18]. Patients may still ask for prescriptions or buy these supplements over the counter, and may even be sure that they work when their osteoarthritis is only taking its natural course, due to regression to the mean, or the placebo effect [9]. Clinicians should discourage patients who ask to be treated with these preparations [18], but since neither of these supplements has been proven harmful, there is no reason clinicians should strongly object if patients think the supplements are beneficial and are willing to pay for them out of pocket [6].

## ACKNOWLEDGMENT

We thank Kali Tal for her editorial suggestions.

## REFERENCES

1. Barnes MB, Bloom B. Complementary and alternative medicine use among adults and children: United States, 2007. Natl Health Stat Report 2008;12:1–9.
2. Bekelman JE, Li Y, Gross CP. Scope and impact of financial conflicts of interest in biomedical research: a systematic review. JAMA 2003;289:454–65.
3. Bijlsma JW, Knahr K. Strategies for the prevention and management of osteoarthritis of the hip and knee. Best Pract Res Clin Rheumatol 2007;21:59–76.
4. Clegg DO, Reda DJ, Harris CL, Klein MA, O'Dell JR, Hooper MM, Bradley JD, Bingham CO III, Weisman MH, Jackson CG, et al. Glucosamine, chondroitin sulfate, and the two in combination for painful knee osteoarthritis. N Engl J Med 2006;354:795–808.
5. Conrozier T, Vignon E. Die Wirkung von Chondroitinsulfat bei der Behandlung der Hüftgelenksarthrose: eine Doppelblindstudie gegen Placebo. Litera Rheum 1992;14:69–75.
6. Felson DT. Chondroitin for pain in osteoartyhritis. Ann Intern Med 2007;146:611–12.
7. Felson DT. Developments in the clinical understanding of osteoarthritis. Arthritis Res Ther 2009;11:203.
8. Fransen M, Agaliotis M, Nairn L, Votrubec M, Bridgett L, Su S, Jan S, March L, Edmonds J, Norton R, et al. Glucosamine and chondroitin for knee osteoarthritis: a double-blind randomised placebo-controlled clinical trial evaluating single and combination regimens. Ann Rheum Dis 2015;74:851–8.

9. Krogsboll LT, Hrobjartsson A, Gotzsche PC. Spontaneous improvement in randomised clinical trials: meta-analysis of three-armed trials comparing no treatment, placebo and active intervention. BMC Med Res Methodol 2009;9:1.
10. McAlindon TE, Biggee BA. Nutritional factors and osteoarthritis: recent developments. Curr Opin Rheumatol 2005;17:647–52.
11. McAlindon TE, LaValley MP, Gulin JP, Felson DT. Glucosamine and chondroitin for treatment of osteoarthritis: a systematic quality assessment and meta-analysis. JAMA 2000;283:1469–75.
12. Nüesch E, Trelle S, Reichenbach S, Rutjes AW, Tschannen B, Altman DG, Egger M, Jüni P. Small study effects in meta-analyses of osteoarthritis trials: meta-epidemiological study. BMJ 2010;341:c3515. doi:10.1136/bmj.c3515.
13. Reichenbach S, Sterchi R, Scherer M, Trelle S, Bürgi E, Bürgi U, Dieppe PA, Jüni P. Meta-analysis: chondroitin for osteoarthritis of the knee or hip. Ann Intern Med 2007;146:580–90.
14. Richey F, Bruyere O, Cucherat M, Henrotin Y, Reginster JY. Structural and symptomatic efficacy of glucosamine and chondroitin in knee osteoarthritis: a comprehensive meta-analysis. Arch Intern Med 2003;163:1514–22.
15. Sawitzke AD, Shi H, Finco MF, Dunlop DD, Bingham CO III, Harris CL, Singer NG, Bradley JD, Silver D, Jackson CG, et al. The effect of glucosamine and/or chondroitin sulfate on the progression of knee osteoarthritis: a report from the glucosamine/chondroitin arthritis intervention trial. Arthritis Rheum 2008;58:3183–91.
16. Sawitzke AD, Shi H, Finco MF, Dunlop DD, Harris CL, Singer NG, Bradley JD, Silver D, Jackson CG, Lane NE, et al. Clinical efficacy and safety of glucosamine, chondroitin sulphate, their combination, celecoxib or placebo taken to treat osteoarthritis of the knee: 2-year results from GAIT. Ann Rheum Dis 2010;69:1459–64.
17. Scarpignato C, Lanas A, Blandizzi C, Lems WF, Hermann M, Hunt RH, for the International NSAID Consensus Group. Safe prescribing of non-steroidal anti-inflammatory drugs in patients with osteoarthritis—an expert consensus addressing benefits as well as gastrointestinal and cardiovascular risks. BMC Med 2015;13:55.
18. Singh JA, Noorbaloochi S, MacDonald R, Maxwell LJ. Chondroitin for osteoarthritis. Cochrane Database Syst Rev 2015;1:CD005614.
19. Towheed TE, Maxwell L, Anastassiades TP, Shea B, Houpt JB, Welch V, Hochberg MC, Wells G. Glucosamine therapy for treating osteoarthritis. Cochrane Database Syst Rev 2005, Updated 2009;2:CD002946.
20. Trelle S, Reichenbach S, Wandel S, Hildebrand P, Tschannen B, Villiger PM, Egger M, Jüni P. Cardiovascular safety of non-steroidal anti-inflammatory drugs: network meta-analysis. BMJ 2011;342:c7086.
21. Vlad SC, LaValley MP, McAlindon TE, Felson DT. Glucosamine for pain in osteoarthritis: why do trial results differ? Arthritis Rheum 2007;56:2267–77.
22. Wandel S, Jüni P, Tendal B, Nüesch E, Villiger PM, Welton N, Reichenbach S, Trelle S. Effects of glucosamine, chondroitin, or placebo in patients with osteoarthritis of hip or knee: network meta-analysis. BMJ 2010;341:c4675.

23. Zhang W, Moskowitz RW, Nuki G, Abramson S, Altman RD, Arden N, Bierma-Zeinstra S, Brandt KD, Croft P, Doherty M, et al. OARSI recommendations for the management of hip and knee osteoarthritis. Part II: OARSI evidence-based, expert consensus guidelines. Osteoarthritis Cartilage 2008;16:137–62.
24. Zhang W, Nuki G, Moskowitz RW, Abramson S, Altman RD, Arden NK, Bierma-Zeinstra S, Brandt KD, Croft P, Doherty M, et al. OARSI recommendations for the management of hip and knee osteoarthritis. Part III: changes in evidence following systematic cumulative update of research published through January 2009. Osteoarthritis Cartilage 2010;18:476–99.

CHAPTER 14

# Exercise, Sport, and Joint Pain

*Mira Meeus, Dorien Goubert, Suzie Van Noten, and John Nijs*

Many different conditions can lead to painful joints, including osteoarthritis, rheumatoid arthritis, bursitis, gout, strains, sprains, and other injuries. Joint pain is extremely common, and is becoming even more prevalent, as people are growing older. Depending on the source, knee, neck, low back, shoulder, and hip pain are the most common, but joint pain can affect any part of the body, from ankles and feet to shoulders and hands, and can be widespread or generalized as well, like, for example, in fibromyalgia and chronic fatigue syndrome.

Despite the fact that different conditions may lead to joint pain, different joints can be afflicted, and different pain mechanisms may be responsible (nociceptive pain, inflammatory pain, central sensitization pain), physical activity and exercise are frequently encountered as a central component in the treatment of patients with chronic joint pain.

## EFFECTS OF EXERCISE THERAPY

The clinical benefits of physical activity and exercise therapy are obvious in different chronic pain populations, as reported in several Cochrane reviews.

Moderate-to-high-intensity resistance training seems to improve multidimensional function, pain, tenderness, and muscle strength in women with fibromyalgia. Low-quality evidence suggests that women with fibromyalgia can safely perform moderate-to-high-resistance training [3]. Also, 8 weeks of aerobic exercise seem efficacious for improving pain in women with fibromyalgia [3].

For patients with osteoarthritis, land-based therapeutic exercise provides short-term benefit in terms of reduced pain [6]. Based on the evidence, aerobic capacity training combined with muscle strength training is recommended as routine practice in patients with rheumatoid arthritis [7].

The type of activity or exercise program generally does not really matter. For chronic musculoskeletal pain, positive effects are found after walking therapy, aerobic exercise therapy, yoga, aquatic exercise, resistance training, etc. [10].

Although positive effects are found for long-term activity or exercise programs, there are also increasing amounts of studies reporting adverse effects of exercise. More specific, it seems that often the acute response to one bout or a short-term exercise intervention is adverse in patients with chronic musculoskeletal pain. Patients often complain of pain exacerbations, increased pain sensitivity, bad recovery, etc.

## RESPONSE TO ACUTE EXERCISE: EXERCISE-INDUCED HYPOALGESIA VERSUS HYPERALGESIA

Besides the beneficial long-term effects of training programs, acute exercise bouts are sometimes used to lower the pain sensitivity. This phenomenon is called exercise-induced hypoalgesia and has been largely investigated in the past years (see meta-analysis [15]). In healthy subjects, it seems that different types of exercise can induce a hypoalgesic effect [15].

However, in patients with chronic joint pain, the effect of an acute bout of exercise is less straight forward because both hypoalgesic and hyperalgesic responses have been reported [11, 14]. In chronic fatigue syndrome, fibromyalgia and chronic whiplash-associated disorders, for example, both aerobic and isometric exercise, seem to decrease pain thresholds and increase temporal summation of pain [11, 13, 14,

18, 19]. In contrast, hypoalgesic effects were noticed in patients with rheumatoid arthritis [13], chronic shoulder pain [11], chronic low back pain [14], etc.

So, it seems that the response to an acute bout of exercise is varying between different chronic musculoskeletal pain conditions. It is assumed that those patients with a dominant picture of central sensitization (= hyperexcitability and thus hypersensitivity of the central nervous system) are the patients with malfunctioning endogenous pain inhibition and those who are thus responding worse to an exercise bout.

In contrast to the centrally sensitized patients at the extreme end of the musculoskeletal pain continuum, other chronic joint pain conditions are more localized/structural. Think, for example, about those suffering from rheumatoid arthritis, osteoarthritis, chronic shoulder or low back pain, etc. Although neuroplastic changes may occur because of continuous noxious stimulation, central sensitization seems to be present only in subgroups of these populations. That is why contradictory findings may be observed in these patients.

Besides the heterogeneity in pain mechanisms between the different subgroups (varying between low to high sensitivity), the type of exercise may also cause different responses. Preliminary evidence, based on very heterogeneous research questions and designs, seems to indicate that nonspecific exercises, like general aerobic training [1, 13, 14] or strength training of nonafflicted body parts [11], can have pain-relieving effects in patients with a more localized/structural chronic pain complaint by reducing pain sensitivity in the affected tissues. This is indicative for a normal activation of endogenous pain regulatory mechanisms, and is supported by the findings of increased pain thresholds and decreased temporal summation both at symptomatic and asymptomatic places [11, 13, 14].

On the other hand, specific training, meaning exercising painful body parts, does not always activate brain-orchestrated analgesia either in the exercising muscle or at distant locations. Contraction of painful muscles failed to activate segmental as well as plurisegmental pain inhibitory mechanisms in shoulder myalgia patients [11]. Possibly, the lack of heterotopic pain inhibition could result from a ceiling effect, that is, an inability to further recruit pain inhibitory mechanisms that are already activated at baseline due to the spontaneously ongoing pain [8]. Bear in mind that exercising painful body parts may enhance local sources of nociception and lead to further peripheral sensitization (see further). Clinically, this is reflected in an increase in pain intensity up to 2 hours after specific strength training [1].

In conclusion, while in healthy participants almost all types of acute exercise reduce perception of experimentally induced pain, the size and direction of the effects for chronic pain conditions depend on the type of medical condition being studied and the type or the specificity of the exercise [15].

## MECHANISMS OF EXERCISE-INDUCED HYPOALGESIA

Although the exact mechanisms behind exercise-induced hypoalgesia are not yet completely unraveled, it is thought that it is likely caused by a combination of factors. The contribution of different mechanisms would depend on the type, duration, intensity, etc. of the exercise [15, 16].

Perhaps, the most widely considered mechanism is the activation of the endogenous opioid system during exercise. Exercise of sufficient intensity and duration results in the release of peripheral and central β-endorphins, which have been associated with changes in pain sensitivity. However, the mixed results in humans and animal studies suggest the existence of non-opioid-dependent exercise-induced hypoalgesia. The opioid mechanism and other possible mechanisms have been the topic of numerous studies and have been extensively described in different overview papers. Therefore, interested readers are referred to these papers [15, 16]. We restrict this part to listing up the different contributing mechanisms. Besides the release of β-endorphins and opioids, the release of cortisol, catecholamines, growth factors, etc. have also been suggested to take part in the phenomenon of exercise-induced hypoalgesia. Exercise may also activate the stress response and gate control mechanisms by activation of, for example, muscle afferents. Or, since some stimuli inherent to exercise may serve as pain stimuli, exercise may stimulate (supra)spinal nociceptive inhibitory mechanisms orchestrated by the brain like in the conditioned pain modulation paradigm. Furthermore, exercise-related changes in heart rate and blood pressure may cause pain modulation, via the baroreceptor reflex, and these two mechanisms share similar brain stem nuclei, neurotransmitters, and neuropeptides. Also, the motor cortex is stimulated during exercise, which contributes to the activation of endogenous pain modulatory systems. Lastly, exercise may cause distraction and increased body awareness for other afferent stimuli (sweating, heart beats, etc.) (for reviews, see [10] and [16]).

## MECHANISMS OF EXERCISE-INDUCED HYPERALGESIA

In the absence of complete understanding of the mechanisms of exercise-induced hypoalgesia, mechanisms underlying exercise-induced hyperalgesia remain unknown, but have been suggested to be caused by abnormal descending inhibition and/or excessive activation of muscle nociceptive afferents [19]. We are talking about the immediate effects of exercise and not about delayed onset of muscle soreness, which is completely different and a far better understood phenomenon.

Activation of nociceptive afferents is indeed inherent to exercise. Many different modes, intensities, and durations of exercise can induce pain in healthy people and in patients. Possible sources of nociception include elevated intramuscular pressure during exercise, release of noxious biochemical, accumulation of metabolites, and deformation or straining of tissue (for review, see[5]). Importantly, some studies suggest dose–response effects [5]. In more vigorous exercise, there is a greater release of inflammatory mediators and cytokines, lactate, increase in oxidative stress, etc., which can (further) excite peripheral nerves. This is also the reason why very intensive exercise is also likely to cause increased pain sensitivity in healthy controls immediately after the effort.

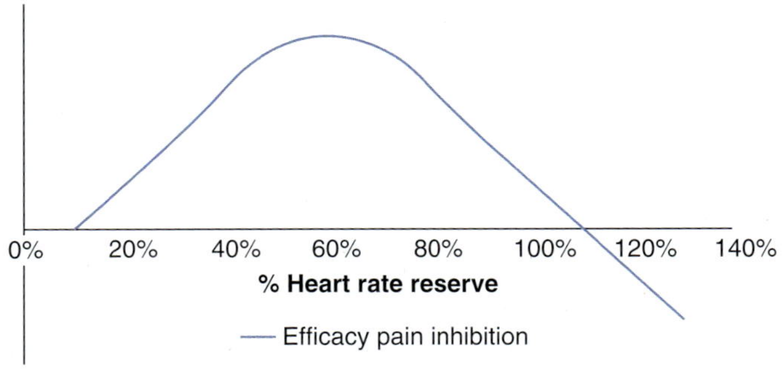


**FIGURE 14-1** Possible relation between exercise intensity and efficacy of immediate pain inhibition.

Probably, the dose–response relation is an inverse U-shaped graph (Fig. 14-1) when it comes to the efficacy of endogenous pain inhibition. It seems that the exercise has to reach a certain intensity (50–70% of heart rate reserve) or duration to activate pain dampening, but too intensive exercise can cause the inverse.

Despite the fact that too intensive exercise can lead to pain in healthy people as well, it seems that in those with chronic joint pain, the acute response to exercise is rather determined by the pain condition/mechanism than by the exercise modalities.

In the more localized chronic pain populations, this is the case for specific exercises (of the afflicted body part), probably because of the ceiling effect [8], as discussed above, and the mechanical strain and buildup of metabolites may explain the transient amplification of pain [1]. Central pain inhibition is, however, working, since it does get activated in response to nonspecific exercises [1, 11].

In those with a dominant picture of central sensitization, there is, however, a failing of pain inhibition during any type of exercise [11, 18].

The background of failing endogenous pain inhibition remains to be unraveled. Based on the hypothetical mechanisms behind exercise-induced hypoalgesia, there have been studies evaluating the association between cardiovascular parameters and pain inhibition during exercise in patients with fibromyalgia [9]. Only a reduced blood flow in the muscle could be observed during static contraction, but differences in heart rate or blood pressure increases were not present and thus probably not related to altered pain modulation. Baroreceptor activation in response to exercise did not result in the typical anti-nociception in patients with chronic low back pain at rest, in contrast to healthy controls [4]. Reduced parasympathetic reactivation during recovery from exercise was associated with the dysfunctional exercise-induced analgesia in patients with chronic fatigue syndrome (Van Oosterwijck et al., unpublished data). Poor recovery of diastolic blood pressure in response to exercise, with blood pressure remaining elevated, is associated with reductions of pain following exercise in patients with chronic fatigue syndrome, suggesting a role for the arterial baroreceptors in explaining dysfunctional exercise-induced analgesia in these patients. However, further work is required (and ongoing) to unravel the potential role of baroreceptor activation in endogenous analgesia in response to exercise in chronic pain patients.

Regarding the role of hormones, more research has been conducted. Especially, the dampened stress response to exercise (release of catecholamines and cortisol) might explain the negative response to exercise in patients with fibromyalgia [9]. But far more research is required to assess the role of eventual altered brain perfusion, serotonin activity, opioids, etc. in the negative response to exercise.

So, it is clear that exercise-induced pain is an end product of peripheral and central inhibitory and facilitatory mechanisms, and exercise induces mechanical, thermal, and chemical stress. In conclusion, in case of unaccustomed exercise or in case of failing endogenous pain inhibition, exercise is likely to cause an immediate increased pain sensitivity.

## LONG-TERM RESPONSE

Another confusing finding in chronic joint pain conditions is the contradiction between the acute response to exercise and the long-term response to exercise training/therapy.

Briefly, the long-term response to training is beneficial for all chronic musculoskeletal pain conditions. Also, patients with an adverse acute response to an exercise bout seem to benefit from physical activity or exercise programs in the longer term (see above), probably because of the reconditioning of both peripheral structures (muscles and joints) and descending antinociceptive mechanisms. Peripheral adaptations on the one hand can include increased muscle strength, which may lower the relative workload of the muscle during daily low-force work tasks (= increased reserve capacity of muscle strength in response to strength training) [1].

But, even more important is the retraining of the brain-orchestrated endogenous pain inhibition. This assumption is supported by the positive relationship between levels of physical activity and brain activity in the posterior cingulate cortex and the dorsolateral prefrontal cortex, involved in top-down modulation of pain, suggesting that physically active persons may regulate pain differently than those who are less active. Regions previously implicated in pain regulation were positively associated with physical activity, while brain regions implicated in the sensory/discriminative aspects of pain processing were negatively related to physical activity, both in healthy controls and in patients with fibromyalgia. Having fibromyalgia patients categorized into high and low physical activity, subgroups revealed greater responses in pain regulatory regions and lesser responses in sensory regions for those with higher self-reported physical activity [12].

Furthermore, it seems that local muscle strength and local pressure pain thresholds are increased after 10 weeks of specific strength training (of the painful muscle). But also the pain thresholds of a pain-free reference muscle increased in response to specific strength, indicating a general effect of physical activity on pain sensitivity [1], and thus indicative of an amelioration of centrally mediated pain modulation, besides peripheral adaptations in muscles and joints.

Finally, animal research data suggest that regular exercise reduced pain by activation of opioid receptors in the descending inhibitory pathways and peripheral opioid receptors (in muscles). But which opioid receptors and the exact locations are yet unclear. Likewise, the effects of exercise on the sympathetic nervous system, cardiovascular system, and motor nervous system might also contribute to the analgesia [5].

## PITFALLS AND CHALLENGES

First of all, and possibly the biggest threat, is the fact that especially immediate effects may determine future exercise behavior and adherence to exercise interventions. Indeed, the first phase of exercise programs is prone to dropouts. So, although exercise-induced hyperalgesia is limited in time, it may have huge effects on longer term, partly mediated by the perceptions and beliefs of the patients. People often interpret pain as an indicator of a physiological problem or bodily harm. Therefore, attributing pain to exercise may lead people to believe they should stop exercising and/or avoid similar exercise in the future, comprising therapy compliance. Reduced or abnormal exercise tolerance may consequently lead to fear of movement and avoidance of certain activities. This may thus lead to further disuse, deconditioning, and further lowering of exercise tolerance [20]. This vicious circle is an important therapy barrier and compromises therapy compliance. So, the risks and dangers of exercise in chronic pain patients have to be explored and taken into account during exercise interventions, for instance, by taking the time to discuss the patients' perceptions regarding anticipated outcomes of exercise bouts and the meaning of any pain exacerbations. When using pain neuroscience education prior to exercise therapy, addressing maladaptive beliefs becomes a natural implementation of the reconceptualization of pain.

Secondly, besides the known relation between physical activity levels and endogenous pain modulation (see above), any intervention to improve endogenous pain inhibition in clinical practice remains, however, speculative. At present, any treatment interfering with descending modulation is currently unavailable for clinical use in chronic pain patients. This comes as no surprise, given the lack of insight into the precise mechanisms of malfunctioning of descending pain inhibition in those with central sensitization, including during exercise. These issues should definitely be addressed in further research: how to prescribe activity programs and exercise therapy for chronic pain patients, in which above-mentioned barriers are avoided and in which progressive and careful retraining of the endogenous pain system is possible.

For the moment, therapists are thus confronting a risky balance act of tailoring the exercise program. On the one hand, therapists should account for the dysfunctional response of patients with chronic pain and aberrations in central pain modulation in response to acute exercise, but on the other hand they should try to distract the focus of pain, as pain is not a reliable alarm sign for damage in many chronic pain patients and hypervigilance for pain should not be encouraged.

## TRAINING ADVICES

Since exercise therapy programs appear beneficial for all chronic pain and even useful for restoring endogenous pain inhibitory mechanisms, the question is no longer "to exercise or not to exercise?" but "how to exercise?"

The specifics of the exercise regimen likely matter less than the way in which exercise is prescribed and taught and the supportiveness of the environment. If you can get your patients moving, they will typically feel better eventually. The key to effective exercise prescription for chronic pain is identifying and promoting strategies that facilitate actual participation in exercise [10]. Therefore, a comprehensive biopsychosocial assessment is necessary to recognize the dominant pain mechanisms, identify possible biomechanical deficits, understand the patients' beliefs and perceptions, evaluate the psychological readiness, unravel possible barriers, etc.

Afterward, appropriate education is necessary. Education can "prime" the patient before starting with the exercise programs. By explaining concepts of central pain processing and the relation with physical activity, the relevance of beliefs and perceptions, the real meaning of pain in case of chronic pain, effects of exercise etc., a lot of inappropriate and pain facilitating beliefs can be altered and their readiness and participation can be enhanced.

Hence, exercise therapy for patients with chronic pain should not apply principles of cardiac or pulmonary rehabilitation. Instead, exercise therapy in these patients should include education about the neurophysiology of pain and central sensitization to reconceptualize the meaning of pain, followed by the identification of an appropriate baseline and goal setting. This baseline level of function should be achievable, so that the patient can start with a success experience. Baseline setting can be performed in a pain-contingent way, meaning that a safe and conservative baseline is determined based on some pain-controlled trials before the start of the exercise therapy. Afterward, a safe and realistic rate of progression is negotiated with the patient. The rate of progression is based on predetermined quota per day, independent of the pain. This means that a time-contingent approach should be used to replace the control of activity from pain (that is not reliable) to a rational process and to enhance self-efficacy. In any case, the patient should experience a success during exercise, and therefore, gentle, individually tailored activity or exercise programs are necessary with emphasis on prevention of symptom flares (eventually with other medical support), in order not to strengthen further catastrophic thinking about exercise and pain. Subsequently, the grading phase included grading of the exercise bouts using a time-contingent approach. This type of exercise therapy accounts for our current understanding of chronic pain neuroscience [10, 17].

Specific guidelines for training formats for patients with chronic joint pain are lacking, but evidence is mounting for aerobic exercise at low levels at which the patient can be successful. Low-level exercise is also more likely to be more conducive to adherence and less likely to provoke symptoms. Patients' preferences should shape the program, but various exercises should be integrated [5].

In those with more localized chronic joint pain complaints or even in those with generalized complaints with local deficits (e.g., muscle weakness), research points out the benefits of more specific training [1, 5]. Possibly, this is not the first step in the training program, and patients should be "primed" first, as explained above.

It is, for example, shown that when comparing general fitness training with more specific strength training in patients with chronic neck pain, specific strength training is the most efficacious in reducing pain and increasing pain thresholds in the longer term, with a lasting effect after cessation of the training. But in the short term, specific strength training indeed increases pain and reduces pain thresholds, whereas general training did not [1]. So, although the acute effects are only short term, even minor decreases in pain may be a motivating factor for persons with severe pain to overcome barriers to exercise, and augmented fitness in response to general fitness training may increase overall health in the long term. Therefore, it seems important to give the patient proper education about the expected effects, emphasizing that the pain is not the consequence of damage and that these exacerbations are only short lasting and occur during the beginning of the training period, but reduce from session to session during the entire intervention period [1].

To activate endogenous pain inhibition to counter the local pain increase, it is probably good to vary sufficiently in exercises and combine both general fitness training with the more specific strength training, especially in the beginning period of the training. Moreover, an important aim of exercise therapy is to train the brain, besides training the musculoskeletal system. The fact that a 2-minute specific training period gives the same pain reduction and increase of both local and distant pain thresholds, compared with a 12-minute specific training period, underlines the fact that a big part of the pain reduction is due to changes in central pain processing, since a 12-minute training period is more efficacious in enhancing muscle performance [2].

## CONCLUSIONS

Overall, exercise appears to have consistent and positive benefits for a multitude of chronic pain conditions. The biggest challenge is that many chronic pain patients show, however, an acute adverse response to exercise. Comprehensive insight in the biopsychosocial profile, the dominant pain mechanisms, and the possible therapy barriers is, therefore, necessary to start the delicate task of exercise prescription. Depending on the type of chronic pain, individually tailored exercises will be more general or specific, but it is always important to give proper education to the patients and address the perceptions and beliefs of the patient to achieve the desired results: pain reduction and reconditioning of both peripherals structures if necessary and even more important of the brain-orchestrated endogenous pain inhibition.

## REFERENCES


1. Andersen LL, Kjaer M, Søgaard K, Hansen L, Kryger AI, Sjøgaard G. Effect of two contrasting types of physical exercise on chronic neck muscle pain. Arthritis Rheum 2008;59:84–91.
2. Andersen LL, Saervoll CA, Mortensen OS, Poulsen OM, Hannerz H, Zebis MK. Effectiveness of small daily amounts of progressive resistance training for frequent neck/shoulder pain: randomised controlled trial. Pain 2011;152:440–6.
3. Busch AJ, Webber SC, Richards RS, Bidonde J, Schachter CL, Schafer LA, Danyliw A, Sawant A, Dal Bello-Haas V, Rader T, Overend TJ. Resistance exercise training for fibromyalgia. Cochrane Database Syst Rev 2013;12:CD010884.
4. Chung O, Bruehl S, Diedrich L, Diedrich A, Chont M, Robertson DY. Baroreflex sensitivity associated hypoalgesia in healthy states is altered by chronic pain. Pain 2008;138:87–97.
5. Cook DB. Pain. In: Ekkekakis P, editor. Routledge handbook of physical activity and mental health. Routledge: New York; 2013. p. 357–410.
6. Fransen M, McConnell S, Hernandez-Molina G, Reichenbach S. Exercise for osteoarthritis of the hip. Cochrane Database Syst Rev 2014;4:CD007912.
7. Hurkmans E, van der Giesen FJ, Vliet Vlieland TP, Schoones J, Van den Ende EC. Dynamic exercise programs (aerobic capacity and/or muscle strength training) in patients with rheumatoid arthritis. Cochrane Database Syst Rev 2009;4:CD006853.
8. Jensen KB, Kosek E, Petzke F, Carville S, Fransson P, Marcus H, Williams SC, Choy E, Giesecke T, Mainguy Y, et al. Evidence of dysfunctional pain inhibition in Fibromyalgia reflected in rACC during provoked pain. Pain 2009;144:95–100.
9. Kadetoff D, Kosek E. The effects of static muscular contraction on blood pressure, heart rate, pain ratings and pressure pain thresholds in healthy individuals and patients with fibromyalgia. Eur J Pain 2007;11:39–47.
10. Kroll HR. Exercise therapy for chronic pain. Phys Med Rehabil Clin N Am 2015;26:263–81.
11. Lannersten L, Kosek E. Dysfunction of endogenous pain inhibition during exercise with painful muscles in patients with shoulder myalgia and fibromyalgia. Pain 2010;151:77–86.
12. McLoughlin MJ, Stegner AJ, Cook DB. The relationship between physical activity and brain responses to pain in fibromyalgia. J Pain. 2011;12:640–51.
13. Meeus M, Hermans L, Ickmans K, Struyf F, Van Cauwenbergh D, Bronckaerts L, De Clerck LS, Moorken G, Hans G, Grosemans S, Nijs J. Endogenous pain modulation in response to exercise in patients with rheumatoid arthritis, patients with chronic fatigue syndrome and comorbid fibromyalgia, and healthy controls: a double-blind randomized controlled trial. Pain Pract 2015;15:98–106.
14. Meeus M, Roussel NA, Truijen S, Nijs J. Reduced pressure pain thresholds in response to exercise in chronic fatigue syndrome but not in chronic low back pain: an experimental study. J Rehabil Med 2010;42:884–90.
15. Naugle KM, Fillingim RB, Riley JL III. A meta-analytic review of the hypoalgesic effects of exercise. J Pain 2012;13:1139–50.

16. Nijs J, Kosek E, Van Oosterwijck J, Meeus M. Dysfunctional endogenous analgesia during exercise in patients with chronic pain: to exercise or not to exercise? Pain Phys 2012;15:ES205–13.
17. Nijs J, Meeus M, Cagnie B, Roussel NA, Dolphens M, Van Oosterwijck J, Danneels L. A modern neuroscience approach to chronic spinal pain: combining pain neuroscience education with cognition-targeted motor control training. Phys Ther 2014;94:730–8.
18. Van Oosterwijck J, Nijs J, Meeus M, Van Loo M, Paul L. Lack of endogenous pain inhibition during exercise in people with chronic whiplash associated disorders: an experimental study. J Pain 2012;13:242–54.
19. Vierck CJ Jr, Staud R, Price DD, Cannon RL, Mauderli AP, Martin AD. The effect of maximal exercise on temporal summation of second pain (windup) in patients with fibromyalgia syndrome. J Pain 2001;2:334–44.
20. Vlaeyen JW, Linton SJ. Fear-avoidance and its consequences in chronic musculoskeletal pain: a state of the art. Pain 2000;85:317–32.

CHAPTER 15

# Analgesic WHO Ladder: Is It Appropriate for Joint Pain? From NSAIDs to Opioids

*Pascale Vergne-Salle and Pierre Beaulieu*

## ANALGESIC LADDER

### Origin and Present Form

In 1986, the World Health Organization (WHO) presented the analgesic ladder as a framework that physicians could use when developing treatment plans for cancer pain [22]. It recommends treating pain based on severity (WHO) (Fig. 15-1). Although it was first proposed for the treatment of cancer-related pain, the WHO pain ladder was soon extrapolated to chronic nonmalignant pain. The WHO proposed the analgesic ladder following the recommendations of an international group of experts. The document was translated into 22 different languages and has served as a catalyst for increasing awareness around the world of the importance of treating pain in cancer patients [20].

The WHO document gives five simple recommendations for the correct use of analgesics to make the prescribed treatments effective: (1) oral administration of analgesics, (2) administration at regular intervals, (3) prescription according to pain intensity as evaluated by a scale of intensity of pain, (4) dosing of pain medication adapted to the individual, and (5) prescription with a constant concern for detail.

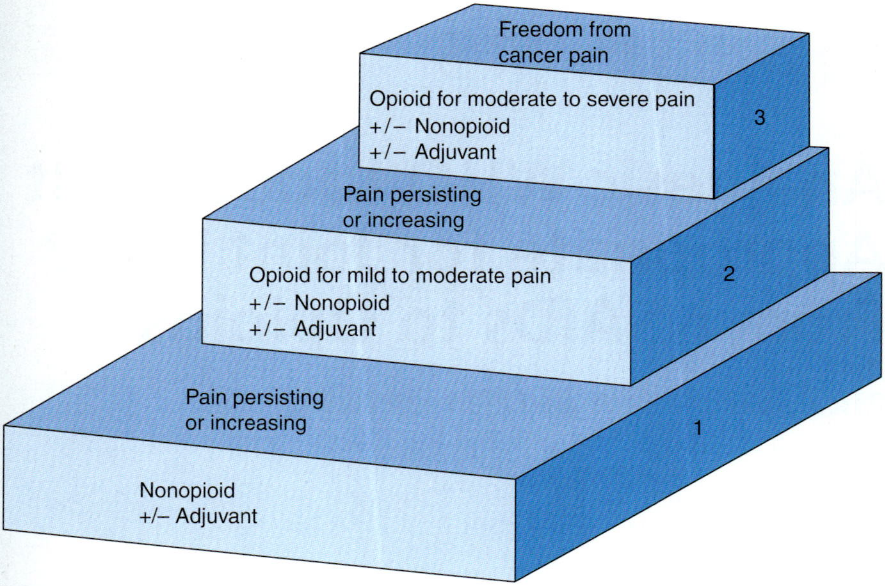


**FIGURE 15-1** WHO analgesic ladder. (World Health Organization [22].)

In the analgesic ladder, non-opioid analgesics (acetaminophen or nonsteroidal anti-inflammatory drugs) are used for mild pain (step I), whereas weak opioids (hydrocodone, codeine, tramadol, low-dose oxycodone) are used for moderate pain (step II) and strong opioids (morphine, hydromorphone, high-dose oxycodone, fentanyl, methadone) are used for severe pain (step III). A more recent but less known WHO classification categorizes analgesics as non-opioids, opioids, coanalgesics (antidepressants, anticonvulsants, ketamine, local anesthetics), or adjuvants (steroids, muscle relaxants, bisphosphonates) [2]. Adjuvant analgesics can be combined with analgesics for the treatment of pain of any severity, depending on the nature of pain; these drugs are also recommended to calm fears and anxiety.

Several authors have proposed modifications to the WHO pain ladder in recent years, because of developing scientific evidence. Eisenberg et al. [5] proposed to eliminate weak opioids for the treatment of cancer pain, because low doses of strong opioids have been shown to provide better and faster pain relief, with greater patient satisfaction [14]. Invasive procedures should be considered at any stage, as an alternative or an adjunct to pharmacotherapy. Vargas-Schaffer [20] proposed to keep steps I–III unchanged and add a fourth step for managing the crises of chronic pain, comprising nerve block, epidurals, patient-controlled analgesia pump, neurolytic block therapy, and spinal stimulators. The treatment should also be adapted to the nature and acuteness of pain, using a step up approach for chronic pain, nonmalignant pain, and cancer pain and a step down approach for acute pain, chronic pain without control, and acute crises of chronic pain.

Although evidence is still limited, there is proof that pain is better controlled, with fewer adverse effects, when using a combination of diverse classes of analgesics [3]. Therefore, when clinicians select the most appropriate analgesics for a given patient, they should combine various analgesics with different mechanisms of action for a better pain relief.

## Acetaminophen

Acetaminophen, also known as paracetamol (*N*-acetyl-para-aminophenol), has analgesic and antipyretic properties and has superior tolerance than NSAIDs, making it appropriate for widespread use in patients. Despite many years of use worldwide and numerous studies, acetaminophen mechanism of action is still uncertain. However, Mallet et al. [12] suggested that the activity of acetaminophen would require a multistep process involving the activity of the endocannabinoid system through supraspinal $CB_1$ receptors, which would in turn reinforce the activity of the bulbospinal serotonergic descending (inhibitory) pathways.

Acetaminophen is recommended as first-line therapy to treat mild-to-moderate pain because of the rarity of toxicity and adverse effects when used at therapeutic doses. Recent evidence and most guidelines recommend a maximal daily dose of 3200 mg when acetaminophen is used for more than 10 days in patients with risk factors for toxicity and 2600 mg in patients with other risk factors (polypharmacy, advanced age, alcohol abuse, liver impairment). When used to treat acute pain of less than 10-day duration, the traditional 4000 mg maximal daily dose can be used. When acetaminophen is administered on a chronic basis, frequent monitoring of liver function tests should be done to avoid liver toxicity.

## Nonsteroidal Anti-Inflammatory Drugs

Nonsteroidal anti-inflammatory drugs (NSAIDs) and selective cyclooxygenase-2 inhibitors (coxibs) are indicated for the treatment of inflammatory diseases or for the treatment of acute pain. Coxibs are as effective as standard NSAIDs in the management of pain. The administration of NSAIDs with morphine is usually associated with a morphine-sparing effect and in some situation (postoperative pain) with a reduction in side effects: less nausea and vomiting, less sedation, but no effect on the incidence of pruritus, urinary retention, or respiratory depression.

Unfortunately, NSAIDs and coxibs are associated with potentially serious side effects that restrain their utilization. It is important to remember that the duration of treatment, the dose administered, and the age of the patient are crucial in producing unwanted effects: the longer the administration, the bigger the dose; and the older the patients are, the more deleterious effects are reported. NSAIDs, including coxibs, are contraindicated in patients with gastrointestinal, renal, cardiac (angina, cardiac failure), or cerebrovascular disease (transient ischemic events or stroke). Coxibs in particular should be used with caution in patients suffering from hypertension, dyslipidemia, diabetes, and in smokers. Finally, a short course of treatment at the lowest efficacious dose is highly recommended.

## Opioids

As indicated earlier, opioids should be used for the treatment of pain of moderate or severe intensity. Treatment should be initiated with a low dose and increased progressively based on analgesic response and tolerability. Responses to various opioids can vary depending on the patient and type of pain. Opioid rotation can be done when pain does not respond to a specific opioid. When prescribing an opioid, it is always important to first evaluate the risk of medication abuse and diversion and then frequently reassess these issues.

# A New Rational Taxonomy

## Existing Classification of Analgesics

Analgesics can be categorized based on different criteria, including severity of pain, type of pain, therapeutic classes of analgesics (e.g., antidepressants, anticonvulsants), mechanisms of action, or a combination of different criteria. Several classifications have been proposed.

Apart from the first classification of analgesics known as the WHO pain ladder (see above), in which treatment is based on pain severity, the most commonly used and clinically relevant classification of analgesics is based on clinical efficacy, for example, multipurpose, neuropathic pain, bone pain, and musculoskeletal pain [10]. The pitfall of this type of classification is the evolving knowledge on analgesic efficacy of various drugs, which would require frequent modifications to the classification.

Analgesics are also categorized based on their original therapeutic class and indication (e.g., antidepressants, anticonvulsants, muscle relaxants, antiarrythmics). This categorization can often be misleading because it might imply that either all drugs from the class have analgesic properties or all drugs from the same class have similar mechanisms of action, neither of which is true. It can also be misleading to patients, who may believe that they are prescribed an antidepressant to treat depression.

Rather than classifying analgesics based on their clinical efficacy or therapeutic class, they can be classified, called mechanistic approaches, by dividing analgesics depending on which pain mechanism they act on or even on the molecular targets. According to Marchand [13], the most appropriate analgesic can then be determined based on the specific mechanism of the patient's pain, for example, nociceptive (somatic, visceral, inflammatory) or neuropathic (complex regional pain syndrome, peripheral and central neuropathic pain, spinal cord injury, functional pain). In contrast to Marchand [13], Costigan and Woolf [4] have divided pain mechanisms into peripheral sensitization, ectopic discharge, sympathetically maintained pain, central sensitization, and reduced inhibition or increased transmission. Moreover, each mechanism is further divided in various molecular targets of analgesics.

### New Mechanistic Classification

Lussier and Beaulieu [9] have proposed a taxonomy of analgesics inspired by previously existing classifications and based mainly on mechanisms of analgesia (Table 15-1). It completely eliminates the term *adjuvant analgesic* and *coanalgesics* and considers them all as analgesics, on the same level as non-opioids and opioids. Furthermore, investigational drugs can be easily added to the classification based on their mechanism of action, which should eliminate the need for frequent modifications to the taxonomy with evolving knowledge.

## JOINT PAIN

In rheumatology, the strategy of joint pain management is not univocal. It will depend on many criteria, including the acute or chronic state of pain. Joint pains are heterogeneous and related to different diseases, especially in terms of pathophysiology. On the other hand, pain management includes both symptomatic and background treatments. In chronic joint pain such as osteoarthritis, inflammatory rheumatic diseases, microcrystalline arthritis, and fibromyalgia, symptomatic treatment is not systematically based on the WHO analgesic ladder. Although joint pain is traditionally considered to be nociceptive, some patients describe aspects of their pain as neuropathic. Within a pain syndrome, heterogeneity between patients in the predominant mechanism of pain is expected and it should lead to therapeutic adaptation.

### Pain Management in Acute Joint Pain

In 2015, the therapeutic goal was to quickly reduce acute pain to improve patient's comfort and to avoid anxiety, sleep disturbance, and cognitive dysfunction, which are risk factors for chronic pain. Effective analgesia allows faster return to normal life, including going back to work.

In acute articular pain, the severity of pain may justify starting immediately with a weak or strong opioid to reduce pain quickly and to switch later for a non-opioid analgesic if the pain becomes tolerable.

TABLE 15-1 **Mechanistic Taxonomy of Analgesics**

| |
|---|
| **Antinociceptive Analgesics** |
| Non-opioids |
| Acetaminophen (paracetamol) |
| NSAIDs |
| Opioids |
| Cannabinoids |
| **Antihyperalgesics** |
| NMDA antagonists |
| Gabapentinoids (gabapentin, pregabalin) |
| Levetiracetam |
| Lamotrigine |
| Nefopam |
| Nitrous oxide |
| Coxibs |
| **Modulators of Descending Inhibition or Excitation** |
| Tricyclic antidepressants |
| SNRIs |
| SSRIs |
| $\alpha_2$-adrenergic agonists |
| **Modulators of Peripheral Transmission/Sensitization** |
| Local anesthetics |
| Carbamazepine |
| Oxcarbazepine |
| Topiramate |
| Capsaicin |
| **Mixed: Antinociceptive Analgesics and Modulators of Descending Inhibition or Excitation** |
| Tramadol |
| Tapentadol |
| **Other** |
| Calcitonin |
| Bisphosphonates |

*Abbreviations*: Coxibs, selective cyclooxygenase-2 inhibitors; NMDA, *N*-methyl-D-aspartate; NSAIDs, non-steroidal anti-inflammatory drugs; SNRIs, serotonin-norepinephrine reuptake inhibitors; SSRIs, selective serotonin reuptake inhibitors.

*Source*: From Lussier D, Beaulieu P. Toward a rational taxonomy of analgesics. In: Beaulieu P, Lussier D, Porreca F, Dickenson AH, editors. Pharmacology of pain. Seattle: IASP Press; 2010. p. 27–40.

Two other criteria have to be considered when choosing the analgesic treatment: the management of incident acute pain related to disease progression and the prevention of induced pain. In the first situation, many inflammatory rheumatic diseases are characterized by more intense painful flare-ups, real breakthrough pain. For breakthrough pain, a fast-acting analgesic treatment should be considered with information and patient education. In rheumatoid arthritis (RA), painful flare-ups could lead to prescribe a step I or II analgesic (see above) or NSAIDs during the day or evening. Induced pains are pain triggered by movements, physiotherapy, or nursing care. These pains could be prevented with patient participation and education. A step I, II, or III analgesic could be proposed to a patient with osteoarthritis before walking or before physiotherapy. The treatment should be adjusted according to its efficacy and tolerance. The analgesic strategy must take into account the schedule of pain and the analgesic drug pharmacokinetic, especially in induced pain.

## Pain Management in Chronic Joint Pain

In chronic articular pain, the mechanistic approach is probably more appropriate for an effective management of pain. The treatment should be based on pain mechanisms: mechanical nociceptive pain, inflammatory nociceptive pain, neuropathic pain, and both nociceptive and neuropathic pain. A better characterization of pain and its mechanisms are required before prescribing analgesic drugs.

### Inflammatory Rheumatic Diseases

Pain related to inflammatory rheumatic diseases is complex with both acute flares and multifactorial chronic pain with an impact on daily life. Analysis of pain clinical features allows to choose an optimal strategy. Different ways are available to estimate disease activity in RA: night pain, morning stiffness, disease activity score (DAS) 28 for RA, ankylosing spondylitis activity score (ASDAS) for spondyloarthritis, erythrocyte sedimentation rate, or C-reactive protein measurement. In inflammatory nociceptive pain, optimal pain treatments are NSAIDs and steroids. In the absence of contraindications, NSAIDs constitute the first-line pharmacological treatment of symptomatic spondyloarthritis [21]. In RA, steroid therapy has symptomatic effects on joint pain and swelling and structural effects. Steroids are recommended early in the course of the disease, in combination with a disease-modifying antirheumatic drug (DMARD), in a small cumulative dosage and for a short duration. The treatment is targeted at obtaining a remission or minimal disease activity in every patient, with the goal of preventing progression of structural damage and the development of disabilities. Follow-up should be provided at short intervals (every 1–3 months) as long as the disease is active. Treatment adjustments are in order in patients who fail to improve within 3 months or to achieve treatment target within 6 months [7]. In patients with inadequate response, biological therapy may be considered (tumor necrosis factor alpha [TNF-α] antagonist, abatacept, tocilizumab, rituximab). Biological therapies have proven efficacy on joint pain [17]. They could be considered as antinociceptive analgesics. However, the add-on therapy with step I or II analgesics is sometimes necessary for better management of chronic articular pain and to decrease breakthrough pain. Indeed, despite an optimal treatment with biological therapy in combination with a DMARD, chronic generalized pain may persist, and it is not always related to the severity and activity of the underlying disease. Among 22,795 patients with RA from Europe and the United States, most of them reported dissatisfaction with arthritis pain management [19]. In some RA patients, pain was due to sequelae after structural joint damage with mechanical nociceptive component such as in osteoarthritis. In such cases, step I to III analgesics have the potential to reduce pain, in combination with local treatments (corticosteroid or hyaluronic acid intra-articular injections) or arthroplasty. Although inflammation contributes to pain in RA, it may not be the only factor. As in other chronic pain states, emotional and cognitive disorders may influence pain perception and cause pain facilitation. When they are identified, psychotherapy, cognitive behavioral therapy, and antidepressants may be useful. In RA patients, few studies have demonstrated hyperalgesia, allodynia, and enhanced pain sensitivity in a widespread distribution (joint and nonjoint sites), indicative of the involvement of the central nervous system [16]. Continuously increased nociceptive inputs could lead to peripheral and subsequently long-lasting central sensitization, giving rise to chronic, persistent pain, stress-related features, behavioral symptoms, fatigue, and mood disorders. Recent data reported at the European League Against Rheumatism (EULAR) congress have demonstrated that about 20% of patients have a positive painDETECT questionnaire indicative of neuropathic pain phenotypic similarities and central sensitization. Glial cells, pro-inflammatory cytokines, and chemokines may contribute to pain sensitization [8]. The relationship between inflammation, psychosocial factors, and peripheral and central pain processing is intricately entwined. The future challenges are to better understand the different pain mechanisms in inflammatory arthritis, to establish pain phenotyping tools, and to study centrally acting analgesic drugs' efficacy.

## Osteoarthritis

Osteoarthritis (OA) is a major cause of pain in elderly patients who are very often polymedicated and present with numerous comorbidities that must be considered when choosing an analgesic. The most frequent treatments are step I and II analgesics, NSAIDs, and local treatments (steroids and hyaluronic acid injections). Step II analgesics and NSAIDs are not always well tolerated, and sometimes despite these treatments, patients have persistent pain. The WHO therapeutic step-by-step approach should theoretically lead to a step III analgesic prescription according to the persistence and severity of pain.

The Osteoarthritis Research Society International (OARSI) developed in 2014 up-to-date, patient-focused, evidence-based, expert consensus guidelines for the management of knee OA [15]. Appropriate modalities for all individuals included biomechanical interventions, intra-articular steroids, exercise, education, and weight management. Treatments appropriate for specific clinical sub-phenotypes included acetaminophen, capsaicin, NSAIDs (oral and topical), and duloxetine. Treatments of uncertain appropriateness for specific clinical sub-phenotypes included chondroitin, diacerein, glucosamine, intra-articular hyaluronic acid, and opioids. Acetaminophen is little effective in OA [11]. NSAIDs are associated with increased risk of gastrointestinal, cardiovascular, and renal adverse effects and are recommended in individuals without comorbidities.

For opioids, the recommendation is uncertain. Analyses of pain relief found a moderate effect size for codeine over placebo, a small to moderate benefit for oxycodone, and a small benefit for tramadol and morphine over placebo. However, patients receiving opioids were four times as likely as patients receiving placebo to withdraw because of adverse events. Opioid analgesics should be prescribed only for patients with refractory OA pain or with contraindications to the recommended treatments, or patients waiting for orthopedic surgery or when surgery is not possible. Outside the WHO analgesic ladder, topical capsaicin is recommended (superior to placebo for 50% pain reduction). Duloxetine is efficacious and tolerable for chronic pain associated with OA, with 16% of patients withdrawing due to adverse events. This antidepressant is considered more appropriate for individuals with multiple-joint OA and relevant comorbidities. Pain characteristics in OA suggest different underlying mechanisms. Although OA pain is traditionally considered to be nociceptive, some patients describe aspects of their pain as burning or shooting. Heterogeneity between patients in the predominant mechanisms of OA pain may contribute to poor response to conventional treatments. Emerging evidence suggests that pain sensitization plays an important role in pain associated with OA. A recent meta-analysis of 15 studies identified widespread hyperalgesia, spinal hyperexcitability, and conditioned pain modulation, suggesting a degree of sensitization in knee OA, associated with symptom severity [6]. The reversibility of sensitization after total knee arthroplasty suggests an association between peripheral pathology and central changes. The central hyperexcitability may also, in some cases, be present before the development of OA. Future research is needed to identify people with sensitization as a dominant feature and to assess their response to treatments, reducing peripheral and central sensitization or enhancing descending inhibitory activity.

## Microcrystalline Arthritides

Microcrystalline arthritides are common inflammatory arthritis conditions causing morbidity, disability, and poorer quality of life. It is the consequence of deposition of crystals in joints or other tissues characterized by acute episodes of inflammation or less frequent chronic articular pain. The WHO therapeutic step-by-step approach cannot be applied. Optimal treatment requires NSAIDs, colchicine, or steroids based on the EULAR recommendations for calcium pyrophosphate deposition and the third initiative recommendations for gout [18, 23].

### Fibromyalgia

In fibromyalgia (FM), treatment recommendations should be directed at reduction of symptoms and fostering optimal function. Ideal management requires a multimodal approach, active patient participation, and nonpharmacological strategies. Pharmacological treatments may be helpful. Acetaminophen and tramadol analgesics lead only to a modest relief of pain. NSAIDs are often prescribed, but randomized clinical trials show lack of superiority compared with placebo. NSAIDs should be used only in associated conditions such as OA, in the lowest dose, and for the shortest possible period of time, in view of potential serious adverse effects. Although assessment of pain is often high in FM patients and should theoretically lead to a prescription of strong opioids based on the WHO ladder, there is no evidence of efficacy and physicians should consider other treatment options. Unanimously, the German, Canadian, and European guidelines strongly discouraged prescription of strong opioids [1]. The recommended treatments are more often modulators of descending inhibition, such as antidepressants and anticonvulsants.

## IS THE WHO LADDER FOR JOINT PAIN APPROPRIATE?

The WHO ladder is appropriate in chronic nociceptive joint pains. But, in most other cases, it is not appropriate. Many mistakes are induced by the WHO ladder considering in a parallel manner the severity of pain and the presumed efficacy of analgesics. The pathophysiology of joint pain is multiple and complex with different underlying mechanisms. The management of joint pains should consider different points: the acute or chronic state of the disease, the nociceptive and/or neuropathic type of pain, and the emotional, cognitive, or professional components. For example, in rheumatic disease, there are probably various subgroups of patients having different pain phenotypes. Before treatment is initiated, an analysis of clinical features and phenotype of pain are necessary. Therefore, a mechanistic approach to pain treatment is probably more appropriate. Indeed, Lussier and Beaulieu [9] proposed a rational taxonomy based on both pain mechanisms and molecular targets of the analgesics that could be used when treating complex and multifactorial pain syndromes. Concerning chronic joint pain, nociceptive inflammatory pain could be treated by reducing inflammation with steroids or NSAIDs, the noninflammatory nociceptive pain by opioid and non-opioid analgesics, and the neuropathic pain by antidepressants or anticonvulsants, including specific drugs in certain rheumatologic clinical situations (e.g., colchicine in gout) (Fig. 15-2). In conclusion, a different approach from the WHO analgesic ladder allows the physician to treat pain according to clinical reality and avoid being locked in a therapeutic escalation of stronger drugs.

## REFERENCES


1. Ablin J, Fitzcharles MA, Buskila D, Shir Y, Sommer C, Häuser W. Treatment of fibromyalgia syndrome: recommendations of recent evidence-based interdisciplinary guidelines with special emphasis on complementary and alternative therapies. Evid Based Complement Alternat Med 2013;2013:485272.
2. American Society of Anesthesiologists Task Force on Chronic Pain Management, American Society of Regional Anesthesia and Pain Medicine. Practice guidelines for chronic pain management: an updated report by the American Society of Anesthesiologists Task Force on Chronic Pain Management and the American Society of Regional Anesthesia and Pain Medicine. Anesthesiology 2010;112:810–33.
3. Chaparro LE, Wiffen PJ, Moore RA, Gilron I. Combination pharmacotherapy for the treatment of neuropathic pain in adults. Cochrane Database Syst Rev 2012;7:CD008943.
4. Costigan M, Woolf CJ. Pain: molecular mechanisms. J Pain 2000;1:35–44.
5. Eisenberg E, Marinangeli F, Birkhahm J, Paladín A, Varrassi G. Time to modify the WHO analgesic ladder? Pain Clin Update 2005;13:1–4.
6. Fingleton C, Smart K, Moloney N, Fullen BM, Doody C. Pain sensitization in people with knee osteoarthritis: a systematic review and meta-analysis. Osteoarthritis Cartilage 2015;23:1043–56.

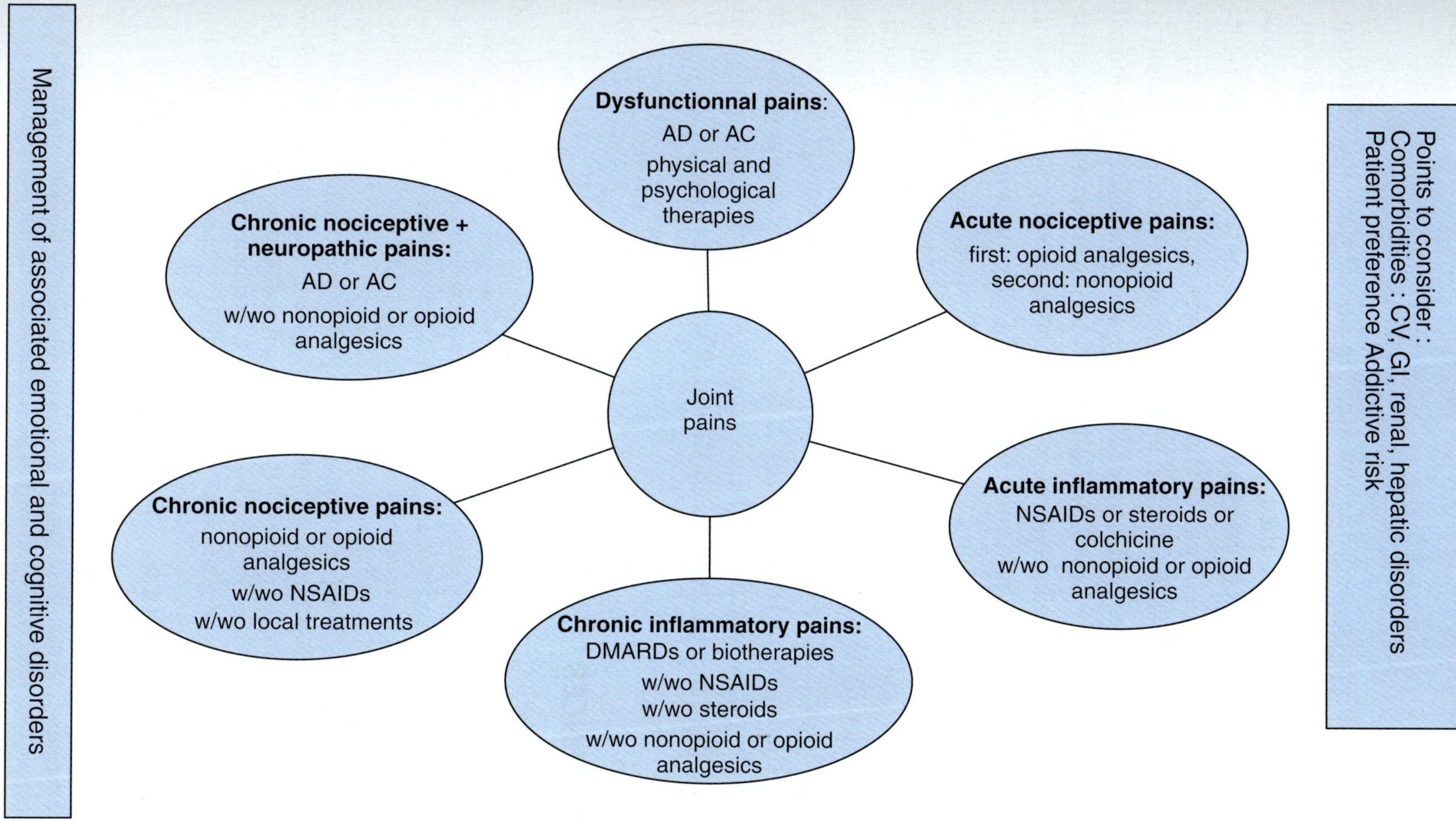


**FIGURE 15-2** Proposed analgesic management for joint pains. AC, anticonvulsants; AD, antidepressants; CV, cardiovascular; DMARDs, disease-modifying antirheumatic drugs; GI, gastrointestinal; NSAIDs, nonsteroidal anti-inflammatory drugs.

7. Gaujoux-Viala C, Gossec L, Cantagrel A, Dougados M, Fautrel B, Mariette X, Nataf H, Saraux A, Trope S, Combe B; French Society for Rheumatology. Recommendations of the French Society for Rheumatology for managing rheumatoid arthritis. Joint Bone Spine 2014;81:287–97.
8. Hess A, Axmann R, Rech J, Finzel S, Heindl C, Kreitz S, Sergeeva M, Saake M, Garcia M, Kollias G, et al. Blockade of TNF-α rapidly inhibits pain responses in the central nervous system. Proc Natl Acad Sci USA 2011;108:3731–6.
9. Lussier D, Beaulieu P. Toward a rational taxonomy of analgesics. In: Beaulieu P, Lussier D, Porreca F, Dickenson AH, editors. Pharmacology of pain. Seattle: IASP Press; 2010. p. 27–40.
10. Lussier D, Portenoy RK. Adjuvant analgesics in pain management. In: Hanks G, Cherny NI, Christakis NA, Fallon M, Kaasa S, Portenoy RK, editors. Oxford textbook of palliative medicine, 4th edition. Oxford: Oxford University Press; 2010. p. 707–34.
11. Machado GC, Maher CG, Ferreira PH, Pinheiro MB, Lin CW, Day RO, McLachlan AJ, Ferreira ML. Efficacy and safety of paracetamol for spinal pain and osteoarthritis: systematic review and meta-analysis of randomised placebo controlled trials. BMJ 2015;350:h1225.
12. Mallet C, Daulhac L, Bonnefont J, Ledent C, Etienne M, Chapuy E, Libert F, Eschalier A. Endocannabinoid and serotonergic systems are needed for acetaminophen-induced analgesia. Pain 2008;139:190–200.
13. Marchand S. The physiology of pain mechanisms: from the periphery to the brain. Rheum Dis Clin North Am 2008;34:285–309.
14. Marinangeli F, Ciccozzi A, Leonardis M, Aloisio L, Mazzei A, Paladini A, Porzio G, Marchetti P, Varrassi G. Use of strong opioids in advanced cancer pain: a randomized trial. J Pain Symptom Manag 2004;27:409–16.
15. McAlindon TE, Bannuru RR, Sullivan MC, Arden NK, Berenbaum F, Bierma-Zeinstra SM, Hawker GA, Henrotin Y, Hunter DJ, Kawaguchi H, et al. OARSI guidelines for the non-surgical management of knee osteoarthritis. Osteoarthritis Cartilage 2014;22:363–388.
16. Meeus M, Vervisch S, De Clerck LS, Moorkens G, Hans G, Nijs J. Central sensitization in patients with rheumatoid arthritis: a systematic literature review. Semin Arthritis Rheum 2012;41:556–67.
17. Nam JL, Ramiro S, Gaujoux-Viala C, Takase K, Leon-Garcia M, Emery P, Gossec L, Landewe R, Smolen JS, Buch MH. Efficacy of biological disease-modifying antirheumatic drugs: a systematic literature review informing the 2013 update of the EULAR recommendations for the management of rheumatoid arthritis. Ann Rheum Dis 2014;73:516–28.
18. Sivera F, Andrés M, Carmona L, Kydd AS, Moi J, Seth R, Sriranganathan M, van Durme C, van Echteld I, Vinik O, et al. Multinational evidence-based recommendations for the diagnosis and management of gout: integrating systematic literature review and expert opinion of a broad panel of rheumatologists in the 3e initiative. Ann Rheum Dis 2014;73:328–35.
19. Taylor P, Manger B, Alvaro-Gracia J, Johnstone R, Gomez-Reino J, Eberhardt E, Wolfe F, Schwartzman S, Furfaro N, Kavanaugh A. Patient perceptions

concerning pain management in the treatment of rheumatoid arthritis. J Int Med Res 2010;38:1213–24.

20. Vargas-Schaffer G. Is the WHO analgesic ladder still valid? Twenty-four years of experience. Can Fam Physician 2010;56:514–17.
21. Wendling D, Lukas C, Paccou J, Claudepierre P, Carton L, Combe B, Goupille P, Guillemin F, Hudry C, Miceli-Richard C, Dougados M; French Society for Rheumatology (SFR). Recommendations of the French Society for Rheumatology (SFR) on the everyday management of patients with spondyloarthritis. Joint Bone Spine 2014;81:6–14.
22. World Health Organization. WHO's pain ladder. Accessed September 9, 2015 at www.who.int/cancer/palliative/painladder/en/.
23. Zhang W, Doherty M, Pascual E, Barskova V, Guerne PA, Jansen TL, Leeb BF, Perez-Ruiz F, Pimentao J, Punzi L, et al. EULAR recommendations for calcium pyrophosphate deposition. Part II: management. Ann Rheum Dis 2011;70:571–5.

CHAPTER 16

# Neuronal Sensitization and Visualization/Monitoring of Joint Pain

*Takahiro Ushida, Tomoko Tetsunaga, Tomohiko Nishigami, Motohiro Kawasaki, Tatsunori Ikemoto, Yoji Osako, and Masashi Izumi*

Joint pain affects people of all generations—from the youth to the elderly. The affected parts of the body and resulting medical conditions may vary according to one's age, level of activity, pre-existing traumas, and history of previous illness. Among adolescents, these problems are normally caused by growth spurts coupled with participation in sports. On the other hand, middle-aged and elderly people commonly experience frozen shoulder or knee osteoarthritis (OA) from the weakening of periarticular muscles and degeneration of intra-articular tissues such as cartilage. Generally, the diagnosis of joint pain consists of a physical diagnosis conducted concurrently with imaging techniques such as X-ray or MRI. Although diagnostic imaging is widely practiced, observations gained through diagnostic imaging do not necessarily reflect the pain experienced by the patient. In a previously conducted epidemiological study, about one-third of individuals with radiographic knee osteoarthritis also had pain. Although epidemiological findings in Japan show that joint deformities detected by diagnostic imaging are more likely to occur as one gets older, it has been discovered that women experience more pain if they have deformities [9] (Fig. 16-1).

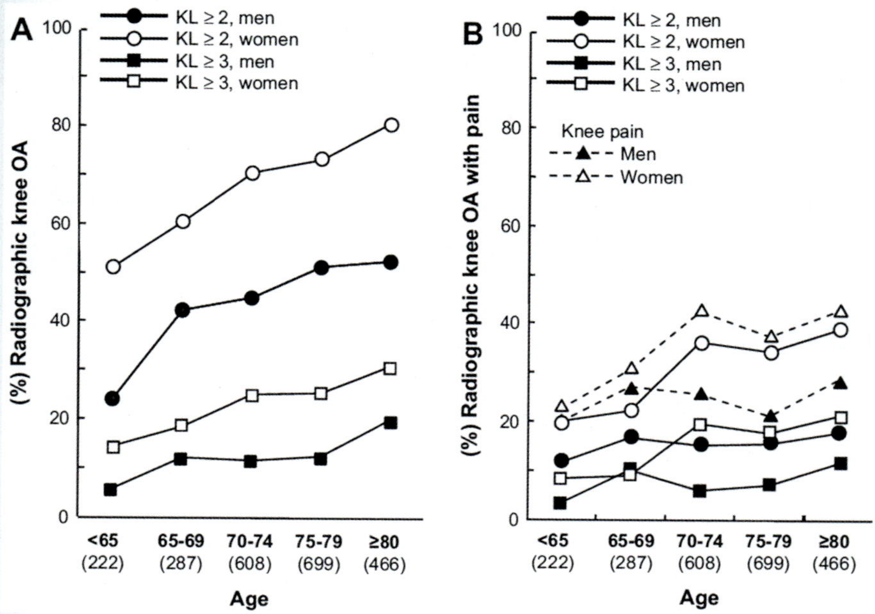


**FIGURE 16-1** Radiographic knee osteoarthritis (OA) and knee pain in the Japanese elderly. The radiographic severity at knees was determined by the Kellgren/Lawrence (KL) grading system. **A:** Percentage of subjects with radiographic knee OA (KL ≥ 2 or KL ≥ 3) in each age stratum (<65, 65–69, 70–74, 75–79, and ≥80). **B:** Percentage of subjects with knee pain and radiographic knee OA (KL ≥ 2 or KL ≥ 3) with pain in each age stratum. The number of subjects in each age stratum is shown in parentheses. (Adapted from Muraki et al. [9].)

In clinical settings, much attention has been placed on local sources of pain in the body (damage of joint cartilage, inflammation of joints, degeneration of periarticular tissues, or even the strength of surrounding tissues) as factors that are responsible for joint pain. Besides these medical examinations conducted in clinics, severe pain experienced by some patients is in fact being alleviated even though we are unable to visualize these disorders, such as joint deformities, through normal radiological imaging technology. On the other hand, there are an extremely large number of cases in which high-level joint deformities do not cause pain or hinder activities of daily life.

Although the clinical significance of a diagnostic imaging assessment of pain, which primarily targets structural factors, is minimal, it is necessary to consider that pain is a neuronal signal that is transmitted to the brain and interpreted as an unpleasant sensation. Since pain is an emotional experience, more focus has been on the research of analyzing joint pain mechanisms based on the study of the nervous system and neurosciences.

Electrophysiological techniques have long been employed to monitor nerve functions, including pain, and neural activity transmitted to the spinal cord through primary afferent fibers from joints has been the subject of detailed analysis. Experiments conducted in the 1980s, which used animals as subjects to determine joint pain through electrophysiological means, have since advanced. Although studies have examined what kind of role the nervous system plays in joint pain transmission, Schmidt et al. [3] reported abnormal discharges from primary afferent fibers due to nociceptive stimuli such as excessive joint extension or bending. They also reported that neural activity similar to joint pain from extension, bending, or stress was recorded in the arthritis model experiment through the use of joint injections, such as kaolin and carrageenan, and that these changes were also recorded in the dorsal horn neurons [11]. In addition, when there is inflammation, the reaction of dorsal horn neurons not only enhances the response to mechanical stimulation in the respective joints, but also transforms and decreases the response threshold of the animal test subjects' ipsilateral distal joints and hind limbs, as well as the enlargement of sensory reception [5]. Applying nociceptive stimulus to joints results in a dorsal root reflex that causes a release of inflammatory neuropeptides in the joints, which worsens arthritis. In studies conducted on rats, this dorsal root reflex occurs bilaterally from Freund's adjuvant-induced chronic arthritis [16]. Furthermore, in the spinal cord, this is caused by glial cell activity, cytokines, or neurotransmitter release. Conducted as a related clinical study, research revealed that before conducting hip arthroplasty for severe hip OA, pain was detected in a wide region that includes 83% of 36 joints. Fourteen percent of the region that experienced pain spread to the lower leg [6] (Fig. 16-2).

When a dorsal root ganglion block was performed, pain relief lasted for 2–3 days in all instances, and in some instances, pain relief lasted for a long period of time [6]. These results suggest that neuronal

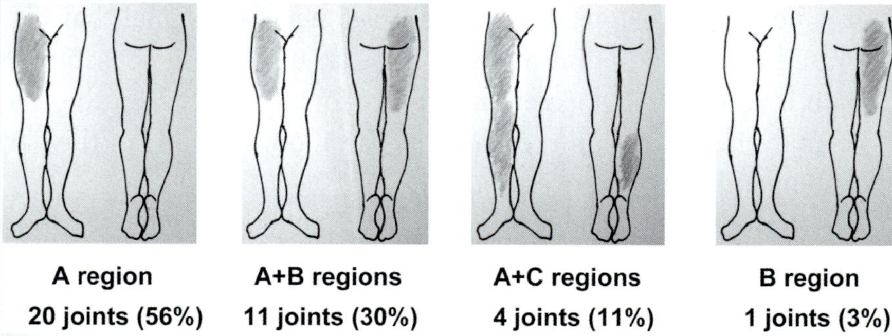


**FIGURE 16-2.** Frequency of the pain regions. **A region:** groin, greater trochanter, and thigh (anterior and lateral); **B region:** buttock and thigh (posterior); **C region:** below knee and leg. (Adapted from Kawada et al. [6].)

sensitizations are underlying factors in chronic joint pain. Graven-Nielsen et al. [4] proposed that this caused patients with knee OA to experience a bilaterally decreased pressure pain threshold. They reported that the decreased pressure pain threshold helped normalize the condition after joint arthroplasty, surmising that peripheral pathological mechanisms affect the spinal cord level and induce pain across a wide region. However, we should mention that 8–23% of those who received joint arthroplasty for knee and other joint problems still experienced pain and we cannot deny the fact that sensitization remained for unknown reasons [7].

Indeed, hypersensitivity and widespread pain on the operated side were found in patients 3 years after total hip arthroplasty [12], suggesting that peripheral and central mechanisms were still active.

Research on joint pain has typically revolved around the use of arthritis models. However, in recent years, studies have also begun to look at medical conditions caused by joint disuse/immobilization. These studies specifically focus on the chronic pain often seen in joint and limb pain caused by immobility or lack of usage of such parts. Okamoto et al. are conducting a study to record the unit potential of primary afferent neurons, which transmit from an animal's joint tissues to its spinal cord, causing a joint contracture. In their research, the animal's joints were inflamed even though they were in a resting state and the same high-frequency discharges were observed from its joints [15]. In addition, it was discovered that when the kinetic load on the joint contracture model animal's contracted limb was increased, the output from the joints increased. Ushida and Willis conducted an electrophysiological study in which they attached an orthopedic cast to the wrist joint contracture model rat for 4 weeks [19]. They observed an enhanced leg withdrawal reflex in this model animal due to nociceptive and heat stimuli. On classifying the neuron type based on the response of the dorsal horn neurons from joint motion and cutaneous stimulation of the affected leg, they reported an increase in the ratio of operation-related neurons in a wide area that responded to nociceptive and nociceptive cutaneous stimulation. At the same time, an increase in the ratio of response to joint motion was also recorded. Furthermore, when the dorsal root ganglions and spinal cords of these animal models were examined through immunohistological techniques, it was discovered that the number of TRPV1-positive and nerve growth factor–positive neurons as well as the large ratio of calcitonin gene-related peptide (CGRP) on the affected side had increased [13]. In addition, through the immobilization of the rat's hind limb, Ohmichi et al. reported a decreased threshold of nociceptive stimuli on both hind limbs and tail. Their study is of great interest as they noticed the activation of microglia in the coccygeal cord and astrocytes after removing the cast following the second-day period [14].

These studies on joint immobilization and other studies on joint tissues highlight that certain functional changes may occur in the spinal cord because of the use of leg casts or non-usage of limbs.

In addition, with regard to the effects of joint immobilization on humans, researchers reported that in cases where immobilization of lower extremity fractures was employed as a course of treatment, it was accompanied by allodynia and other pain that caused difficulty in moving [2].

By attaching an orthopedic cast for 4 weeks to a normal healthy person's upper limbs, allodynia symptoms appeared [18], accompanied by a reduction of the primary somatosensory cortex map correlating with the upper extremities in the brain [8]. In addition, Taniguchi et al. reported that the relative frequency of F waves decreased when upper limbs were fixed in one position for 3 hours [17]. This means that simply not moving our limbs could possibly cause large functional changes in our sensory and motor systems. This also emphasizes that we should place more attention on immobilization as a factor associated with abnormal pains and sensations.

In an fMRI study, pressure stimulation applied to the painful site of OA knees showed activity in the bilateral thalamus, secondary somatosensory cortex (S2), insula, supplementary motor area (SMA), anterior cingulate (ACC), and medial frontal gyrus as well as unilaterally in the right putamen and left amygdala [1]. This activity pattern is markedly different from pain-related activity observed in chronic back pain patients but similar to acute pain activity in normal subjects. This suggests that manifestations of sensitization to joint pain take place through the entire nervous system.

Recently, researchers have begun to recognize central widespread pain and hypersensitivity as important concepts for understanding chronic joint pain. Brain connection network analysis in patients by using the resting state fMRI method has revealed that the Default Mode Network (a set brain region involved in monitoring the internal environment for the detection of salient events) shows greater connectivity to the insular cortex, a brain region known to process evoked pain in individuals suffering from chronic pain conditions such as fibromyalgia [10]. In addition, a functional alteration of the nucleus accumbens and dysfunction of the pain inhibitory system (periaqueductal gray, etc.) results in failure to regulate pain and is a contributor to pain chronicity [20] (Fig. 16-3). Since fibromyalgia is often accompanied by polyarthralgia, it is important to be aware of the underlying central widespread pain and hypersensitivity during therapeutic management.

## ACKNOWLEDGMENTS

Takahiro Ushida would like to thank the late Professor William D. Willis Jr. for mentoring pain research. We would also like to extend our gratitude to Professor Hiroshi Yamamoto, Professor Lars Arendt-Nielsen, and the late Professor Takao Kumazawa for all their kind and valuable advice.

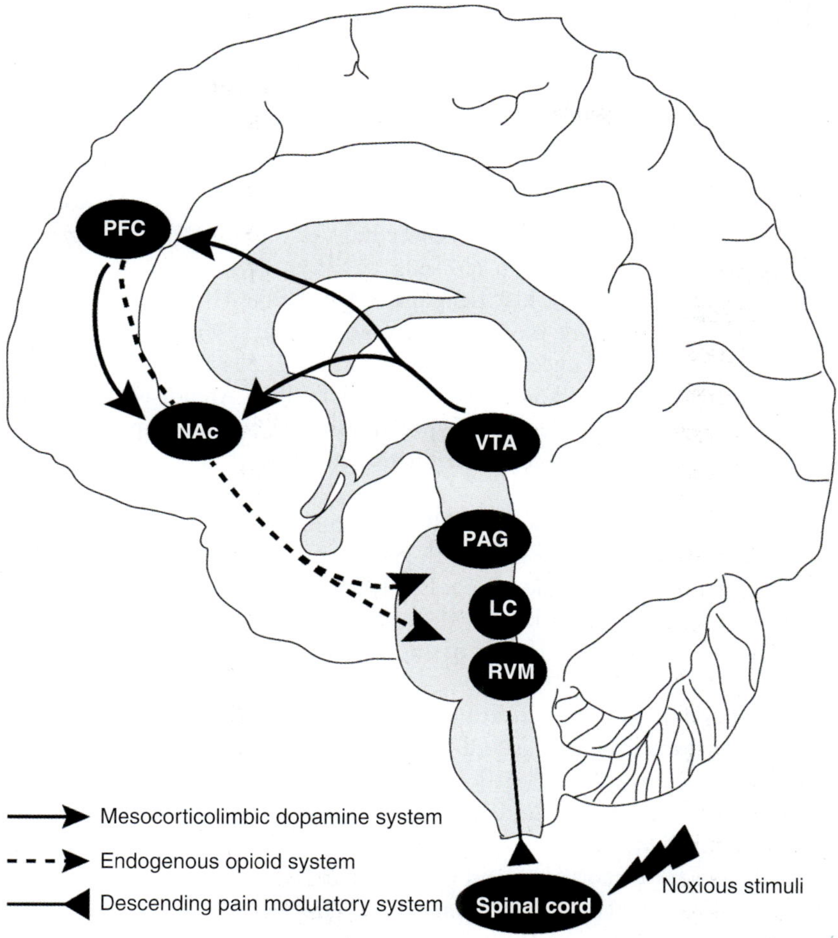


**FIGURE 16-3** Sagittal view of a human brain illustrating a dopamine and opioid system for pain modulation. In this modulation, noxious stimuli activate the ventral tegmental area (VTA), resulting in increased dopamine activity in the prefrontal cortex (PFC) and nucleus accumbens (NAc), that is, stimulating mesocorticolimbic dopamine system. (The connection between the PFC and NAc is glutamatergic fibers.) Subsequently, the endogenous opioid system is thought to drive and act on the descending pain modulatory system consisting of the periaqueductal gray (PAG), locus ceruleus (LC), and rostroventromedial medulla (RVM) in the brain stem. Consequently, the mesocorticolimbic dopamine system can indirectly modulate nociceptive processing in the spinal cord. The source of opioid peptide acting on the PAG, LC, and RVM has not been defined (hence the dotted line).

## REFERENCES

1. Baliki MN, Geha PY, Jabakhanji R, Harden N, Schnitzer TJ, Apkarian AV. A preliminary fMRI study of analgesic treatment in chronic back pain and knee osteoarthritis. Mol Pain 2008;4:47.
2. Butler S, Nyman M, Gordh T. Immobility in volunteers transiently produces signs and symptoms of complex regional pain syndrome. In: Devor M, Rowbotham M, Wiesenfeld-Hallin Z, editors. Proceedings of the 9th World Congress on Pain. Seattle: IASP Press; 2000. p. 657–60.
3. Coggeshall RE, Hong KA, Langford LA, Schaible HG, Schmidt RF. Discharge characteristics of fine medial articular afferents at rest and during passive movements of inflamed knee joints. Brain Res 1983;272:185–8.
4. Graven-Nielsen T, Wodehouse T, Langford RM, Arendt-Nielsen L, Kidd BL. Normalization of widespread hyperesthesia and facilitated spatial summation of deep-tissue pain in knee osteoarthritis patients after knee replacement. Arthritis Rheum 2012;64:2907–16.
5. Grubb BD, Stiller RU, Schaible HG. Dynamic changes in the receptive field properties of spinal cord neurons with ankle input in rats with chronic unilateral inflammation in the ankle region. Exp Brain Res 1993;92:441–52.
6. Kawada T, Ushida T, Ikeuchi M, Kawakami T, Yamanaka N, Ikemoto T, Tani T, Komatu M. Clinical study of hip joint referred pain (Japanese). Pain Res 2006;21:127–32.
7. Lingard EA, Sledge CB, Learmonth ID, GROUP KO. Patient expectations regarding total knee arthroplasty: differences among the United States, United Kingdom, and Australia. J Bone Joint Surg 2006;88:1201–7.
8. Lissek S, Wilimzig C, Stude P, Pleger B, Kalisch T, Maier C, Peters SA, Nicolas V, Tegenthoff M, Dinse HR. Immobilization impairs tactile perception and shrinks somatosensory cortical maps. Curr Biol 2009;19:837–42.
9. Muraki S, Oka H, Akune T, Mabuchi A, En-yo Y, Yoshida M, Saika A, Suzuki T, Yoshida H, Ishibashi H, et al. Prevalence of radiographic knee osteoarthritis and its association with knee pain in the elderly of Japanese population-based cohorts: the ROAD study. Osteoarthritis Cartilage 2009;17:1137–43.
10. Napadow V, LaCount L, Park K, As-Sanie S, Clauw DJ, Harris RE. Intrinsic brain connectivity in fibromyalgia is associated with chronic pain intensity. Arthritis Rheum 2010;62:2545–55.
11. Neugebauer V, Schaible HG. Evidence for a central component in the sensitization of spinal neurons with joint input during development of acute arthritis in cat's knee. J Neurophysiol 1990;64:299–311.
12. Nikolajsen L, Kristensen AD, Thillemann TM, Jurik AG, Rasmussen T, Kehlet H, Jensen TS. Pain and somatosensory findings in patients 3 years after total hip arthroplasty. Eur J Pain 2009;13:576–81.
13. Nishigami T, Osako Y, Ikeuchi M, Yuri K, Ushida T. Development of heat hyperalgesia and changes of TRPV1 and NGF expression in rat dorsal root ganglion following joint immobilization. Physiol Res 2013;62:215–9.

14. Ohmichi M, Ohmichi Y, Ohishi H, Yoshimoto T, Morimoto A, Li Y, Sakurai H, Nakano T, Sato J. Activated spinal astrocytes are involved in the maintenance of chronic widespread mechanical hyperalgesia after cast immobilization. Mol Pain 2014;10:6.
15. Okamoto T, Atsuta Y, Shimazaki S. Sensory afferent properties of immobilised or inflamed rat knees during continuous passive movement. J Bone Joint Surg Br 1999;81:171–7.
16. Rees H, Sluka KA, Lu Y, Westlund KN, Willis WD. Dorsal root reflexes in articular afferents occur bilaterally in a chronic model of arthritis in rats. J Neurophysiol 1996;76:4190–93.
17. Taniguchi S, Kimura J, Yamada T, Ichikawa H, Hara M, Fujisawa R, Shimizu H, Tani T. Effect of motion imagery to counter rest-induced suppression of F-wave as a measure of anterior horn cell excitability. Clin Neurophysiol 2008;119:1346–52.
18. Terkelsen AJ, Bach FW, Jensen TS. Experimental forearm immobilization in humans induces cold and mechanical hyperalgesia. Anesthesiology 2008;109:297–307.
19. Ushida T, Willis WD. Changes in dorsal horn neuronal responses in an experimental wrist contracture model. J Orthop Sci 2001;6:46–52.
20. Vachon-Presseau E, Martel MO, Roy M, Caron E, Albouy G, Marin MF, Plante I, Sullivan MJ, Lupien SJ, Rainville P. Acute stress contributes to individual differences in pain and pain-related brain activity in healthy and chronic pain patients. J Neurosci 2013;33:6826–33.

CHAPTER 17

# Joint Pain in Childhood

*Kerstin Gerhold, Jacqui Clinch, and Carl L. von Baeyer*

Joint pain is a common complaint in children and adolescents, as detailed below. It frequently leads to visits to primary health care providers, with subsequent referrals to sports medicine specialists, orthopedic surgeons, pediatric rheumatologists, physiotherapists, occupational therapists, and chiropractors. Diseases and disease courses may differ between children and adults. In addition, the developing physiological and musculoskeletal systems within a growing child can present challenges when dealing with pain; the mechanical forces are changing and physiological responses may differ from those seen in adulthood. The brain is constantly remodeling; this in turn can affect processing of and response to pain [11, 33].

Underlying conditions leading to joint pain in children and adolescents are numerous, ranging from acute injuries to chronic conditions due to overuse in athletes, from infections to autoimmune-driven inflammation, and from local benign and malignant bone tumors to systemic malignancies and metabolic diseases (Table 17-1). This chapter outlines noninflammatory and inflammatory joint conditions, including typical pathophysiology, symptoms, diagnostic approaches, and principles of treatment using a few examples.

**TABLE 17-1 Examples of Conditions Possibly Accompanied by Joint Pain in Children and Adolescents**

| Supposed Pathomechanism | Example |
|---|---|
| **Noninflammatory Joint Pain** | |
| Biomechanical conditions | • Hypermobility<br>• Patellofemoral knee pain<br>• Femoral acetabular impingement |
| Developmental disorders | • Legg–Calvé–Perthes disease<br>• Slipped capital femoral epiphysis |
| Overuse conditions | • Osteochondritis dissecans<br>• Wrist overuse injuries in gymnastics<br>• Tennis elbow<br>• Golfer elbow |
| Pain amplification | • Regional<br>– Complex regional pain syndrome<br>• Widespread<br>– Fibromyalgia |
| **Inflammatory Joint Pain** | |
| Infectious-related | • Septic arthritis<br>– Bacterial<br>– Staphylococcal<br>– Streptococcal<br>– *Kingella kingae*<br>– *Mycobacterium tuberculosis*<br>– Fungal<br>– Viruses<br>– Spirochetes<br>– Lyme disease<br>• Immune-reactive<br>– Reactive arthritis<br>– Acute rheumatic fever<br>– Poststreptococcal arthritis |
| Possibly infection-related or unclear | • Transient synovitis of the hip<br>• Vasculitides<br>– Henoch–Schönlein purpura<br>– Kawasaki disease |

TABLE 17-1 **Examples of Conditions Possibly Accompanied by Joint Pain in Children and Adolescents (*continued*)**

| **Supposed Pathomechanism** | **Example** |
|---|---|
| Spectrum of autoimmunity | • Juvenile idiopathic arthritis<br>• Connective tissue diseases<br>– Systemic lupus erythematosus<br>– Juvenile dermatomyositis<br>– Mixed connective tissue disease<br>– Undifferentiated connective tissue disease<br>– Localized scleroderma<br>– Juvenile systemic sclerosis<br>– Sjögren syndrome<br>• Vasculitides<br>– Periarteritis nodosa<br>– ANCA-positive vasculitides |
| Spectrum of autoinflammation | • Arthropathy in inflammatory bowel disease<br>• Sarcoid<br>• Behcet disease<br>• Autoinflammatory bone disorders<br>– Chronic nonbacterial osteomyelitis/chronic recurrent multifocal osteomyelitis<br>– Genetically determined autoinflammatory syndromes |
| **Systemic Diseases with Joint Involvement** | |
| | • Vitamin D deficiency (rickets)<br>• Celiac disease<br>• Cystic fibrosis |
| Metabolic diseases | • Increased uric acid production and gout<br>– Lesch–Nyhan syndrome (primary)<br>– Glycogenosis type I (glucose-6-phosphate dehydrogenase deficiency)<br>– Myelo- and lymphoproliferative disorders<br>• Sphingolipidoses<br>– Gaucher disease<br>– Farber disease<br>– Fabry disease<br>• Mucopolysaccharidoses |

(*continued*)

TABLE 17-1 **Examples of Conditions Possibly Accompanied by Joint Pain in Children and Adolescents**

| Supposed Pathomechanism | Example |
|---|---|
| Hematological disorders | • Hemoglobinopathies<br>– Sickle cell disease<br>– β-Thalassemia<br>• Hemophilia<br>– Hemophilia A |
| **Neoplasms** | |
| Benign juxta-articular tumors of the bone, cartilage, and soft tissues | • Osteoid osteoma<br>• Osteoblastoma<br>• Osteochondroma<br>• Chondroblastoma<br>• Fibrous cortical defect (nonossifying fibroma)<br>• Juvenile fibromatosis<br>• Pigmented villonodular synovitis<br>• Intra-articular/periarticular vascular anomalies |
| Malignant juxta-articular tumors of the bone, cartilage, and soft tissues | – Osteosarcoma<br>– Ewing sarcoma<br>– Fibrosarcoma |
| Primary malignant diseases of the bone marrow with juxta-articular lesions | – Acute lymphoblastic leukemia |

## EPIDEMIOLOGY AND IMPACT OF JOINT PAIN IN CHILDREN AND ADOLESCENTS

Pediatric data defining prevalence and risk factors for joint pain are available for specific joint conditions such as those identified below; however, we are aware of no studies or reviews that summarize epidemiological data for all joint pains as a class, differentiating these from other locations or sources of pain. Musculoskeletal pain is a much more common category for epidemiological studies, but most of these studies do not separate joint pain from other musculoskeletal pains [15].

Nevertheless, some impressions may be gained from reviews and surveys on the epidemiology of pediatric recurrent and chronic pain, and from studies of the impact of obesity on joint pain.

In a study of 569 Norwegian school children aged 10 to 15 years, knee pain was the most frequently reported site by both boys (32%) and girls (29%), followed by back pain (22% and 30%), ankle pain (7% and 12%), and foot pain (8% and 11%) [24]. In a survey of German school children, limb pain (specific joints were not defined) showed an overall 3-month prevalence of 46%, in comparison with headaches (66%) and abdominal pain (48%). The peak age was 13–15 years, and girls reported limb pain more often than boys [21]. The female preponderance is confirmed for many musculoskeletal (and other) recurrent pain conditions starting around puberty [7, 15].

An increasing prevalence with age is clearly evidenced; for example, a study in Finland reported the point prevalence of chronic knee pain as 4% in children between 9 and 10 years of age versus 19% in adolescents between 14 and 15 years of age, with no increase attributed to being overweight. Most children with chronic knee pain were involved in athletic activities [31].

Several other studies have examined musculoskeletal consequences of obesity, providing an indication of normative frequencies of joint pain in their comparison groups. Knee pain was the most common self-reported joint complaint, occurring in 21% of overweight children and adolescents and in 17% of nonoverweight subjects [29]. In a similar comparison, at least one "osteoarticular manifestation" was observed in obese patients (55%) compared with the control group (23%) [10]. Most obese youth (61%) complained of at least one joint hurting more than once per month: Back pain was the most common complaint (39%), followed by foot (26%) and knee (24%) pain [26]. Overall, in adolescents, the short-term prevalence of pain in at least one joint appears to be at least 20% and perhaps as high as 50%. Increasing age, female sex, and obesity are the best-documented factors contributing to joint pain.

Pain-associated disability affects a significant minority of young people with persistent musculoskeletal pain. This includes major restriction in daily life activities and impaired health-related quality of life [15, 16, 20].

About 10% of children and adolescents with chronic pain develop severe comorbid conditions, including sleep disturbance, anxiety, or depression, resulting in social withdrawal and inability to participate in physical exercise, social activities, and school [14]. Health care professionals are often overwhelmed with children and families describing increasing pain and pain-associated disability; this can lead to multiple investigations, polypharmacy, doctor shopping, and finally chronification of symptoms with persistence into adulthood. As a consequence, significant burdens for health and school systems may arise.

## UNDERLYING PATHOLOGIES OF JOINT PAIN

### Noninflammatory Joint Disorders

In school-aged children and adolescents, joint pain of noninflammatory origin is far more common than pain based on inflammation. Biomechanical imbalances between bones, cartilage, tendons, muscles, and the tissues surrounding joints during phases of skeletal growth appear to contribute to joint pain, which is often benign and self-limiting. Other factors including joint laxity (hypermobility), obesity, and co-existing morbidities such as myopathies, skeletal dysplasias, and dystrophies can further compound the imbalance and resulting load through joints.

One example of a rather benign joint condition is patellofemoral knee pain. Although not fully understood, it is believed to be caused by malalignment of the patella relative to the femoral trochlea during the pubertal growth spurt. Vastus medialis obliquus insufficiency and hip weakness may contribute to its development. About 1 in 10 physically active female adolescents are affected [5].

The maturing skeleton is also susceptible to develop potentially disabling conditions such as avascular necrosis. Legg–Calvé–Perthes disease (avascular necrosis of the femoral epiphysis) is based on interruption of the femoral head blood supply; a definite cause is unknown [9]. It develops mostly in children between 4 and 10 years of age; boys are about four times more often affected than girls, and both hips may be sequentially involved in about 10–15% of all cases [9, 17]. Slipped capital femoral epiphysis may compromise the vascular supply to the femoral head and is an important cause of secondary avascular necrosis [12]. Orientation and shape of the proximal femur, the acetabulum, and the epiphysis in combination with obesity and hormonal factors are known to contribute to the risk of slipped capital femoral epiphysis during skeleton growth. Its incidence rate is about 10 per 100,000 children and adolescents per year; patients are usually older, between 10 and 16 years of age [12].

Chronic joint pain may be part of a pain disorder; pain disorders may develop primarily or secondarily to an underlying disease such as juvenile idiopathic arthritis (JIA). The pain may be regional as in complex regional pain syndrome or widespread as in fibromyalgia or widespread musculoskeletal pain.

The pathogenesis of chronic pain disorders is thought to be multifactorial and includes minor injuries or illnesses, significant life changes or psycho-social stress factors, insufficient coping abilities, as well as genetic factors; the child's personality is often described as being mature and perfectionistic [22]. One view holds that widespread or multiple pains reflect a biologically based pain vulnerability that is partly genetically based, is associated with vulnerability to anxiety and depression, and is influenced by environmental factors including stress, injury, and illness [32]. Widespread pain is reported in 2–6% of schoolchildren and adolescents; girls are more often affected than boys. Adolescents with joint hypermobility are at increased risk to develop joint pain as well as widespread pain [6, 15, 22, 30].

## Inflammatory Joint Disorders

Joint pain is a typical symptom of arthritis, the inflammation of the synovial membrane lining the inner wall of the joint capsule of synovial joints, bursae, and tendon sheets. Synovial inflammation arises from direct invasion of viable microbes in septic arthritis, from adaptive immune responses to microbial antigens in reactive or postinfectious arthritis or acute rheumatic fever, or from autoimmune processes in JIA, connective tissue diseases, or vasculitides. Acute arthritides due to infections are much more common than chronic arthritis of autoimmune conditions.

The main cause of septic arthritis is bacterial infections, although infections with viruses, spirochetes, and fungi are observed. Bacterial joint infections are medical emergencies: Joints can quickly suffer irreversible damage as cartilage is destroyed within a few days [9]. In developed countries, the incidence rate of septic arthritis is 10–80 per 100,000 children per year [2].

Infants and toddlers younger than 2 years of age are particularly at risk because the metaphyses of long bones receive an extraordinarily high blood supply during skeletal growth. The blood flow in the capillary bed is slow, and during bacteremia, microbes can migrate through the capillary endothelium, causing secondary metaphyseal infection [3]. The metaphysis is intra-articular in infants, and transphyseal vessels may transmit bacteria from the metaphysis to the joint. Therefore, juxta-articular osteomyelitis can present as septic arthritis in this population [2].

Special types of bacterial joint infections include septic arthritis in several joints in septic children, neonates, or immunocompromised patients [2, 3], tuberculous arthritis, and Lyme disease (see Table 17-1). Reactive arthritis secondary to systemic infections (usually viral or bacterial) in children is common. Joints may become painful and swollen for up to 3 months after upper respiratory, gastrointestinal, or sexually transmitted infections. Typically, the joint symptoms resolve, but occasionally they can continue as the underlying condition leads to a more persistent arthritis.

The most prevalent chronic arthritis in pediatric populations is JIA. Prevalence is estimated at about 100 per 100,000 children and adolescents [23]. JIA is defined as arthritis of unknown etiology that begins before the 16th birthday and persists for at least 6 weeks; other known conditions have to be excluded [18]. Following the revised International League of Associations for Rheumatology classification criteria, JIA subtypes take into account the number of affected joints at onset and during the disease course, extra-articular symptoms such as enthesitis, fever, and rashes including psoriasis of the skin and nails as well as immunological parameters [18].

### Joint Pain Caused by Malignant Diseases

Joint pain of noninflammatory or inflammatory conditions can be mimicked by malignant disorders of the bone marrow, by juxta-articular benign bone tumors such as osteoid osteoma or malignant bone tumors such as osteosarcoma, or by juxta-articular bone metastases due to extraosseous malignancies such as neuroblastomas.

In a retrospective study of 286 children with acute lymphoblastic leukemia, 18.5% of the patients presented with localized joint pain; 50% of them had objective signs of arthritis, most frequently presenting as arthritis in less than five joints (oligoarthritis). The type of arthritis is generally secondary to bone, periosteal, or capsular lesions rather than to direct synovial inflammation [4]. Children with joint involvement had less frequent constitutional symptoms and objective signs of hematological disease such as cytopenias. Almost 70% of patients were initially misdiagnosed with reactive arthritis, osteomyelitis, or JIA. The authors summarized that "physicians evaluating children with joint involvement must always be aware of the possibility of underlying malignancy" [4].

## PAIN CHARACTERISTICS IN NONINFLAMMATORY JOINT DISORDERS

In noninflammatory joint disorders, joint swelling is not the hallmark. Nevertheless, transient and mild joint swelling may appear because of inflammation secondary to mechanical irritation of the synovia. For example, in osteochondritis dissecans, joint swelling often follows physical activity, which is in contrast to inflammatory disorders where swelling is more pronounced in the morning.

In a condition such as patellofemoral knee pain, peripatellar or retropatellar pain in one or both knees after prolonged sitting with flexed knees is characteristic. Pain occurs insidiously during physical activity, particularly walking stairs, squats, and weight-bearing sports. Patients may have the feeling that their knees are giving way because of pain or muscle deconditioning. On examination, the knees are *not* swollen or limited in range of motion. Malalignment of the lower limb such as genu valgum or leg length discrepancy may be present. Suprapatellar pressure during isometric contraction of the quadriceps muscle in full knee extension or pushing the patella toward the trochlea typically provokes the pain [5]. Thigh muscles may be tender and/or weak, but usually not atrophic.

In Legg–Calvé–Perthes disease, limping on and off over days up to weeks is typical. Pain is of variable severity, and in contrast to children with septic arthritis, children with Legg–Calvé–Perthes disease usually bear weight. Because of the innervation of the hip, the pain may radiate to the medial thigh, the buttock, and the knee [9]. On examination, antalgic gait is typical, and the body may lean toward the affected side while standing; the gait may also be stiff in the hip, and the leg is often moved by moving the pelvis and lower back. Ranges of internal rotation and abduction of the affected hip are limited at first; hip flexion and extension are usually in normal ranges [9, 17]. In slipped capital femoral epiphysis, patients limp because of hip, groin, thigh, or knee pain. In the case of an acute slip, they may not be able to bear weight. On examination, the affected hip is held in abduction and external rotation; active and passive internal rotation and adduction are decreased [12].

Constitutional symptoms are not characteristic of idiopathic Legg–Calvé–Perthes disease or slipped capital femoral epiphysis. Secondary musculoskeletal effects, if untreated, can follow Legg–Calvé–Perthes disease and slipped capital femoral epiphysis; these include muscle weakness, atrophy, and lower lumbar discomfort.

In chronic pain disorders, joint pain is severe and often increases over time. If a child develops persistent joint pain with pain-associated disability, then a number of other distressing symptoms are described. Often, pains migrate to involve many joints particularly in load-bearing areas, and in addition to pain within the joints, the young person describes extreme sensitivity to touch over that area (allodynia). The pain is not responsive over the long term to analgesics or nonsteroidal anti-inflammatory drugs. In pain disorders, joint pain may be accompanied by morning stiffness, myalgia, chronic headaches and/or abdominal pain, irritable bowel syndrome, nonrestorative sleep or sleep disturbances, chronic fatigue, anxiety, and depression [22]. On examination, children's behavior often appears incongruent with their reported pain, and they may be able to do exercises they reported as not being possible for them to do. The affected joints are not swollen, and limited range of motion is often not objectifiable. Spontaneous pain or pain on palpation is typically not at the joint line as described for inflammatory joint disorders. Allodynia and touch sensitivity may be present in widespread pain and in complex regional pain syndrome; they do not follow specific dermatomes as described in neuropathic pain due to peripheral nerve injury [7, 8, 22].

In widespread pain, muscles may be somewhat weak and deconditioned because of relieving postures and the lack of physical activity; however, definite decrease in muscle strength and muscle atrophy usually does not occur [1]. In regional pain disorders such as complex regional pain syndrome, muscle atrophy can develop because of complete disuse of the affected extremity.

## PAIN CHARACTERISTICS IN INFLAMMATORY JOINT DISORDERS

Onset of joint pain in septic arthritis due to bacterial infection is usually, but not always, acute [25]. Typically, the pain is severe and present at rest. The child will avoid movement of the joint, and younger nonverbal children may present with pseudoparalysis of the affected extremity because of the severe pain. Eighty percent of septic arthritis occurs in the large joints of the lower extremities, including hips, knees, and ankles [2]. Constitutional symptoms including fever and malaise are characteristic, but occasionally severe pain and constitutional symptoms may be absent, and the child may appear well with only mild joint tenderness on examination [2]. The affected joint is usually erythematous, warm, and swollen. Passive and active movement of the joint is restricted. Inflammation of the hip may cause pain radiating into the knee (hips should be examined if a young person has knee pain), and the hip is often held flexed and externally rotated [9]. In contrast to the severe pain in acute bacterial arthritis, joint pain is not the hallmark in tuberculous joint infection and in Lyme disease [13, 19, 25, 27].

# DIAGNOSTIC APPROACH OF JOINT PAIN IN CHILDHOOD

## General Diagnostic Considerations

A detailed history and careful examination of a child with joint pain are considered to be the most important steps on the way to the diagnosis. However, since children particularly of younger age groups are often not good historians and clinical symptoms are sometimes not consistent or difficult to objectify in the physical examination, it may be challenging to distinguish benign biomechanical conditions because of skeletal growth from rare but potentially disabling or even life-limiting noninflammatory and inflammatory diseases. Common blood tests are frequently not specific or even contributory, but may be helpful to detect systemic inflammation or malignant blood disorders such as leukemia. Specific blood tests may confirm a clinically considered diagnosis such as positive Lyme serology. Guidelines for assessment are available, including a sample interview schedule [7].

In patients with primary or secondary chronic joint pain and pain-associated disability, repetition and addition of diagnostics should be avoided to prevent wrong expectations, delay in rehabilitation, further frustration, and finally aggravation of the pain.

Keeping the age group of the patient in mind as noted above, the following questions may help to guide primary care physicians in their diagnostic approach and further referral or treatment decisions:

- Which joint(s) is (are) affected?
- How did the pain develop—acute or gradual, constant, or intermittent?
- How severe is the joint pain? Is the child limping? Is the child weight-bearing?
- What are the aggravating and alleviating factors? In which situations does the joint pain occur and how long does it last? Does the pain occur at night?
- Is there objectifiable joint swelling or limited range of motion? Is there objectifiable accompanying weakness or atrophy of the joint surrounding muscles?

- Does the child have extra-articular symptoms such as constitutional symptoms, or involvement of other organs such as skin, lymph nodes, lungs, heart, liver, spleen, kidneys, or brain?

## Laboratory Tests

Erythrocyte sedimentation rate (ESR), C-reactive protein (CRP), and complete blood count (CBC) may give the first hints to differentiate between inflammatory and noninflammatory joint disorders. Systemic inflammation with increased ESR >40 mm/h, CRP >20 mg/L, and white blood count (WBC) of >12 per nanoliter is suspicious for the diagnosis of septic arthritis [9, 28]. In contrast, CRP, ESR, and CBC are usually normal in Lyme disease [25]. JIA is a clinical diagnosis; blood tests are needed to exclude other diagnoses such as infectious diseases or malignancies. Elevation of CRP or ESR and detection of antinuclear antibodies, rheumatoid factor, or HLA-B27 do not contribute to confirm the diagnosis. Nevertheless, ESR and CRP may be (mildly) increased in JIA. But, increased ESR, CRP, and/or abnormal CBC should raise the differential diagnosis of malignancy. Normal CBC does not necessarily exclude leukemia [4].

Blood cultures, joint fluid cytology, and bacterial, fungal, and mycobacterial cultures of the joint fluid are strongly recommended if septic arthritis is a differential diagnosis. The joint aspirate should be inoculated into a blood culture bottle to enhance the growth of fastidious organisms such as *Kingella kingae* [2]. Serology to detect underlying infections with microorganisms such as *Bartonella*, *Histoplasma*, *Brucella*, or *Borrelia* and a Mantoux test or interferon-gamma releasing assay to test for tuberculosis may be useful approaches to find rare disease causes [2].

## Imaging Studies

Imaging studies including ultrasound, plain radiography, or magnetic resonance imaging (MRI) may be helpful tools for the diagnostic workup of joint pain.

Ultrasound is a safe and quick method to demonstrate joint effusion and inflammation of the synovia with thickening and increased blood supply.

A plain radiograph does not contribute to the early diagnosis of osteomyelitis or avascular necrosis within the first 7–21 days after disease onset, but it may be helpful to exclude traumatic lesions and benign or malignant bone tumors, or to detect bone changes due to metabolic or other genetic diseases.

An MRI is a sensitive method to find joint effusions and to differentiate between involvement of the synovial membrane of joints, tendons, and bursae, and involvement of bone and soft tissue in inflammatory and noninflammatory conditions. It can capture osteomyelitis and abscesses as well as avascular necrosis at much earlier stages than plain radiographs [9]. The MRI has mainly replaced the bone scan if the site of pain is identified. Bone scans with $^{99}$technetium-labeled radiotracer are a sensitive but unspecific method, since uptake of the radiotracer may be increased in malignancies of the bone, in the area of fractures, and in the area of the growth plate. Nevertheless, a bone scan may be still used if the site of inflammation is unknown, if more than one site of inflammation is expected, or if an MRI is not available [2].

## PRINCIPLES OF TREATMENT OF JOINT PAIN

Treatment may depend on the joint condition: Specific treatment approaches are available for some noninflammatory conditions with structural changes of the joint such as surgical fixation of unstable slipped capital femoral epiphysis [12]. Specific medical treatment is also available for most of the inflammatory joint conditions such as antibiotics for infectious joint diseases [2, 19, 25] or disease-modifying antirheumatic drugs such as methotrexate for autoimmune conditions such as JIA.

Some treatment approaches are independent from the underlying cause of joint pain. Short-term treatment with acetaminophen and/or nonsteroidal anti-inflammatory drugs such as ibuprofen or naproxen may provide pain relief in almost all conditions; however, long-term treatment without re-evaluation of the diagnosis should be avoided, particularly in nondefined conditions.

Physiotherapy is a major approach in all joint conditions that are accompanied by limited range of motion of affected joints or tightness, weakness, deconditioning, or atrophy of muscles; common goals are preservation or re-establishment of normal range of motion of joints, and muscle strengthening and muscle reconditioning. Supportive taping or bracing of affected joints during physical activity may help to overcome joint instability. Firm shoes may be supportive in conditions with malalignment to avoid pain such as in patellofemoral knee pain.

In primary or secondary chronic pain syndromes, multimodal treatment approaches have become standard of care [7, 22]. Multimodal treatment includes education of patients and their families about development and management of chronic pain as a first step. Occupational therapy or physical therapy may be needed for desensitization in children with neuropathic signs such as touch sensitivity and allodynia; intensive physical therapy is used for muscle relaxation and reconditioning in physically inactive children. With psychological treatment, most often cognitive behavioral therapy, patients may be able to develop self-reliance and to implement coping strategies into their daily life. Comorbid conditions such as sleep disturbance, depression, and anxiety may need pharmacotherapy in addition to psychological treatment [7, 22]. The overall goals of treatment are primarily to restore normal social and physical function including body perception; improvement in pain generally follows those improvements.

## CONCLUSION

Joint pain is a frequent complaint in children and adolescents, leading to consultations with physicians and other health care providers.

The range of differential diagnoses is wide. Benign biomechanical conditions due to skeletal growth are typical in school-aged children and adolescents. They usually do not go along with joint swelling, limited range of motion, or muscle atrophy. However, patients with rare noninflammatory and inflammatory joint disorders or systemic diseases with joint involvement have to be identified to avoid potential joint damage, disability, and death. The combination of a complete history, thorough examination, laboratory tests, and imaging studies is usually needed to overcome this challenge. In children and adolescents with more severe or complex conditions, the best approach is referral to an interdisciplinary pain team.

## ACKNOWLEDGMENTS

The authors appreciate the comments of Jennifer N. Stinson, PhD. The authors have no conflicts of interest related to the content of this chapter.

## REFERENCES

1. Anthony KK, Schanberg LE. Assessment and management of pain syndromes and arthritis pain in children and adolescents. Rheum Dis Clin North Am 2007;33:625–60.
2. Arnold JC, Bradley JS. Osteoarticular infections in children. Infect Dis Clin North Am 2015;29:557–74.
3. Bonhoeffer J, Haeberle B, Schaad UB, Heininger U. Diagnosis of acute haematogenous osteomyelitis and septic arthritis: 20 years experience at the University Children's Hospital Basel. Swiss Med Wkly 2001;131:575–81.
4. Brix N, Rosthoj S, Herlin T, Hasle H. Arthritis as presenting manifestation of acute lymphoblastic leukemia in children. Arch Dis Child 2015;100:821–5.
5. Carry PM, Kanai S, Miller NH, Polousky JD. Adolescent patellofemoral pain: a review of evidence for the role of lower extremity biomechanics and core instability. Orthopedics 2010;33:498–507.
6. Castori M, Morlino S, Celletti C, Ghibellini G, Bruschini M, Grammatico P, Blundo C, Camerota F. Re-writing the natural history of pain and related symptoms in the joint hypermobility syndrome/Ehlers–Danlos syndrome, hypermobility type. Am J Med Genet A 2013;161A:2989–3004.
7. Clinch J, Eccleston C. Chronic musculoskeletal pain in children: assessment and management. Rheumatology (Oxford) 2009;84:466–74.
8. Connelly M, Schanberg L. Latest developments in the assessment and management of chronic musculoskeletal pain syndromes in children. Curr Opin Rheumatol 2006;18:496–502.
9. Cook PC. Transient synovitis, septic hip, and Legg–Calvé–Perthes disease: an approach to the correct diagnosis. Pediatr Clin North Am 2014;61:1109–18.
10. De Sa Pinto AL, de Barros Holanda PM, Radu AS, Villares SM, Lima FR. Musculoskeletal findings in obese children. J Paediatr Child Health 2006;42:341–44.

11. Fitzgerald M. The development of nociceptive circuits. Nat Rev Neurosci 2005;6:507–20.
12. Georgiadis AG, Zaltz I. Slipped capital femoral epiphysis: how to evaluate with a review and update of treatment. Pediatr Clin North Am 2014;61:1119–35.
13. Hoffman EB, Allin J, Campbell JA, Leisegang FM. Tuberculosis of the knee 2002;398:100–6.
14. Huguet A, Miró J. The severity of chronic pediatric pain: an epidemiological study. J Pain 2008;9:226–36.
15. King S, Chambers CT, Huguet A, MacNevin RC, McGrath PJ, Parker L, Macdonald AJ. The epidemiology of chronic pain in children and adolescents revisited: a systemic review. Pain 2011;152:2729–38.
16. Malleson P, Clinch J. Pain syndromes in children. Curr Opin Rheumatol 2003;15:572–80.
17. Mazloumi SM, Ebrahimzadeh MH, Kachooei AR. Evolution in diagnosis and treatment of Legg–Calve–Perthes disease. Arch Bone Joint Surg 2014;2:86–92.
18. Petty RE, Southwood TR, Manners P, Baum J, Glass DN, Goldenberg J, He X, Maldonado-Cocco J, Orozco-Alcala J, Prieur AM, et al. International League of Associations for Rheumatology classification of juvenile idiopathic arthritis: second revision, Edmonton 2001. J Rheumatol 2004;31:390–2.
19. Rajakumar D, Rosenberg AM. Mycobacterium tuberculosis monoarthritis in a child. Pediatr Rheumatol Online J 2008;6:15.
20. Roth-Isigkeit A. Pain among children and adolescents: restrictions in daily living and triggering factors. Pediatrics 2005;115:152–62.
21. Roth-Isigkeit A, Thyen U, Raspe HH, Stöven H, Schmucker P. Reports of pain among German children and adolescents: an epidemiological study. Acta Paediatr 2004;93:258–63.
22. Sherry DD. Diagnosis and treatment of amplified musculoskeletal pain in children. Clin Exp Rheumatol 2001;19:617–20.
23. Shiff NJ, Lix LM, Oen K, Joseph L, Duffy C, Stringer E, Tucker LB, Svenson LW, Belisle P, Bernatsky S. Chronic inflammatory arthritis prevalence estimates for children and adolescents in three Canadian provinces. Rheumatol Int 2015;35:345–50.
24. Smedbråten BK, Natvig B, Rutle O, Bruusgaard D. Self-reported bodily pain in schoolchildren. Scand J Rheumatol 1998;27:273–6.
25. Sood SK. Lyme disease in children. Infect Dis Clin North Am 2015;29:281–94.
26. Stovitz SD, Pardee PE, Vazquez G, Duval S, Schwimmer JB. Musculoskeletal pain in obese children and adolescents. Acta Paediatr 2008;97:489–93.
27. Szer IS, Taylor E, Steere AC. The long-term course of Lyme arthritis in children. N Engl J Med 1991;325:159–63.
28. Taekema HC, Landham PR, Maconochie I. Distinguishing between transient synovitis and septic arthritis in the limping child. Arch Dis Child 2009;94: 167–8.
29. Taylor ED, Theim KR, Mirch MC, Ghorbani S, Tanofsky-Kraff M, Adler-Wailes DC, Brady S, Reynolds JC, Calis KA, Yanovski JA. Orthopedic complications of overweight in children and adolescents. Pediatrics 2006;117:2167–74.

30. Tobias JH, Deere K, Palmer S, Clark EM, Clinch J. Joint hypermobility is a risk factor for musculoskeletal pain during adolescence: findings of a prospective cohort study. Arthritis Rheum 2013;65:1107–15.
31. Vahasarja V. Prevalence of chronic knee pain in children and adolescents in northern Finland. Acta Paediatr 1995;84:803–5.
32. von Baeyer CL, Champion GD. Multiple pains as functional pain syndromes. J Pediatr Psychol 2011;36:433–7.
33. Walker SM. Overview of neurodevelopment and pain research, possible treatment targets. Best Pract Res Clin Rheumatol 2014;28:213–81.

# INDEX

Note: Page numbers followed by *f* refer to figures and *t* to tables.

## K



## L



## M



## N



## O